DESCENT & RISING

WOMEN'S STORIES &
THE EMBODIMENT OF THE INANNA MYTH

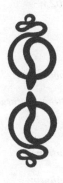

CARLY MOUNTAIN

WOMANCRAFT PUBLISHING

Published by Womancraft Publishing, 2023
www.womancraftpublishing.com

ISBN 978-1-910559-84-0

Descent & Rising is also available in ebook format: ISBN 978-1-910559-83-3

Cover design, interior design and typesetting: lucentword.com

Cover image © Meike Hakkaart

Menstrual cycle illustration: Mimi Mountain

Spiral map and snake icons: Aurora Mountain

Womancraft Publishing is committed to sharing powerful new women's voices, through a collaborative publishing process. We are proud to midwife this work, however the story, the experiences and the words are the authors' alone. A percentage of Womancraft Publishing profits are invested back into the environment reforesting the tropics (via TreeSisters) and forward into the community.

PRAISE FOR
DESCENT & RISING

In this beautifully articulated offering, Carly Mountain takes her place in the lineage of writers honouring the profound significance of the journey of descent as a path of initiation for women. Skillfully and fluidly linking the ancient myth of Inanna with current social, political, ecological and health crises, she includes contemporary women's stories that illustrate an embodied feminine path of healing and awakening to deeper truth and authentic life.

Empowerment through encounter with our deepest wounds and connection to the deep feminine within is an essential task for our troubled times, as we transition towards a re-balancing of feminine and masculine energies in the world. This book serves as an inspiring and timely reminder and a support for all those who find themselves on this path.

Linda Hartley, author of *Servants of the Sacred Dream*, founder of the Institute for Integrative Bodywork & Movement Therapy, and teacher of the Discipline of Authentic Movement

Carly Mountain skilfully guides us on a descent into the wild territory of a woman's psyche and soul. Weaving together the story of the Sumerian goddess Inanna with the author's personal story and those of other women, she maps a distinctly feminine heroic journey – one that honors our depths and brings us to wholeness.

**Mary Reynolds Thompson, author of
Reclaiming the Wild Soul and *A Wild Soul Woman***

Reading Descent & Rising is to be invited into an ancient lineage of feminine wisdom, which for many of us perhaps was forgotten, but as we discover through this rich and insightful book, was never lost. Carly weaves magic as she illuminates the timeless intelligence of one of our oldest goddess myths through the lens of real-life underworld experiences. The result is a wise, warm and engaging companion for those of us who have been through a painfully deep 'underworld' experience, and a sanctuary for those who are being stripped to their core. Let Carly, Inanna and Ereshkigal guide you, step by step, gate by gate, as you descend and discover your very own heroine's journey.

**Alexandra Pope and Sjanie Hugo Wurlitzer, authors of
*Wise Power: discovering the liberating power of menopause
to awaken Authority, Purpose and Belonging***

Descent & Rising offers Inanna's ancient mythology as a captivating foundation for healing and ascension. Carly Mountain's compassionate shares from women around the world are brilliantly woven. Some of us need a merciful nudge to move through the despair that accompanies descent. These stories of women who have resurrected themselves will inspire many women to rise.

Trista Hendren, Creatrix of Girl God Books

Descent and Rising is a summons, a companion and a map to the deep self that is essential in this perilous moment of our personal and planetary history. Carly Mountain has created a masterpiece, seamlessly and sensitively weaving threads of intimate personal narrative with ancient myth, modern science, psychology, poetry, spirituality and more. Through her poetic and compelling prose, I discover myself in the heart of a girl in Kenya fleeing FGM, in the finally free grief cry of a woman in Ireland, in revelations from trauma therapists, neurologists, poets and visionaries. Perhaps the greatest gift that Mountain transmits is an uncanny intimacy with Inanna herself. Here is the companion many of us have longed for as we feel our way through the darkest moments of our lives. I enter these pages alone and emerge rooted in a community of wisdom that not only spans the globe but reaches back in time to the ancestors and forward to those who will come after us, carrying the medicine of these teachings in their cells.

Kim Rosen, author of *Saved by a Poem: The Transformative Power of Words*

In Descent and Rising, Carly Mountain offers us a powerful, in-depth exploration of one of the most important Goddess myths of all time. While thousands of years old, the myth of the Goddess Inanna's descent is startling relevant to our current times, and Mountain breathes new life into our understanding of it, seamlessly weaving together historical facts, critical analysis, and many personal stories drawn from her own life and the lives of other women who have navigated their own descent. A must-read and a sacred companion for any brave woman wishing to dive into the holy darkness of her own self.

Liz Childs Kelly, host of Home to Her podcast, and author of
Home to Her: Walking the Transformative Path of the Sacred Feminine

Permissions

CONTENTS

*To my wonderful Grandma, who sang to me,
and told me magical stories.
I miss you.*

*And to anyone navigating their own descent and rising,
may this myth be a map that helps light the way.*

Opening

From the Great Above Inanna opened her ear to the Great Below.
From the Great Above the goddess opened her ear to the Great Below
From the Great Above Inanna opened her ear to the Great Below.

Diane Wolkstein and Samuel Kramer,
Inanna: Queen of Heaven and Earth

In 2020 the world went quiet. The traffic stopped, the schools closed, people were asked to stay at home. In the absence of the busyness of normal life, we began to open our ears to the great below, the underworld of our personal and collective lives.

I see the story of the heroine's journey unfolding everywhere I look. We are waking up to the ways that we have not been looked after in society and have not looked after others and the Earth. Many of us emerged from the Covid lockdowns not wanting to go back to the way it was before, but not knowing what different would look like either. There is an unshakeable feeling that we don't want to be complicit with the ways we have lived for so long.

Our bodies have started to say no, and we can no longer ignore them.

The new wave of feminism is embodied. It is not just an ideology, it's a physical reality. We want to feel safe when we walk down the street, we want to be heard when we say no, we want pleasure, we want to allow our rage, we want to open to all the feelings we have not admitted. We don't just want change, we are changing. Not only in our thoughts, in our bodies. We are tearing down the old monuments and are discovering in the process, that our own bodies hold the keys to the kingdom. But that's not enough either, we don't want to fill a man's shoes. We want to step, with bare feet, into the wilderness and walk our own path, and we are doing it.

The heroine is one who has started to see the ways in which she has colluded with narratives that no longer serve her, or that maybe never served her. It is an awakening to her-story. I believe that the heroine's path does not lie in new narratives but is sewn into the most ancient ones, and is embedded in our bones, flesh and blood. We are not arriving somewhere new, we are remembering something old: we are rebirthing the heroine from within.

This book is about the importance of stories, how we embody them and how they influence our personal and collective lives. How many stories are we told and do we tell in a lifetime? Stories capture our imaginations, they can inspire and enliven us and have the power to open us up to new worlds and ideas. Many stories also have an underworld – a dark side – that can threaten our sense of self and safety. Some stories narrow our perspective and seek to dominate us. And the trauma held in our bodily stories can trap us in the past, constricting the way we grow. For centuries, stories have been used as a form of control as much as liberation. Our world religions are structured around stories that give us moral codes, guidance on how we should and should not live, teaching what will bring us love, or what can destroy us. Wars have been fought, and continue to be fought, on the basis of these stories.

Mythologies are our most potent and ancient stories, they hold archetypal energies which are alive in us here and now. They can sanction new awakenings and plummet us into layers of feeling and landscapes previously unseen. They hold the power to abolish our blindness, remove the masks from our personas and utterly transform our feelings about ourselves and how we perceive the world. In times of uncertainty, myths may be medicinal, providing much needed guidance. But they are not straightforward. The myths we are craving never come wrapped in the red bow that we ordered. Unlike the lighter stories of life, myths are treacherous and humbling and almost always involve an encounter with grief, shadow and sacrifice. They offer us maps for the most challenging rites of passage we may face in a lifetime and if we survive the journey there is only one guarantee: we will not emerge the same as we entered.

Since I was a young child, I have loved stories. Whilst my brother was always out playing, I could be found with my head in a book or writing. I ate words for breakfast. They absorbed and captivated me. But not all the stories I received shaped me well as a girl, or a woman. Little Red Riding Hood was the first story that really impacted me. At age three I had nightmares about the Big Bad Wolf. Looking back, it was a story that taught me to fear wolf nature and its wildness. But it also taught me that things are not always what they seem, an idea too huge to articulate, but the fear of it was acute. The stories I received about birth also told me to be afraid, that women couldn't cope with pain and that birth might look like lying on my back and screaming to little avail. The stories I was told about sex first came from men, wrapped in jokes, inappropriate and intrusive. Other stories about sex generally emphasised fear of pregnancy and predation, or, conversely, how to be an attractive sexual object for the male gaze. For many years my menstrual cycle was largely unacknowledged and there were no stories to give it meaning. So, like many women before and after me, I forgot the stories of my body. My blood wisdom was like buried treasure on an island called me, that not even I knew about.

Without the stories to symbolise my inner world in the outer world, I paled into the background of his-story. Her-story and, therefore, my story, was not on the map. I was fortunate, in that my parents were gender aware, supportive and encouraged me to be anything I wanted to be. As a girl I was pretty confident, outspoken and unafraid to make myself and my views known. But I, like all my female counterparts, was working against a tide of misogyny and I subconsciously embodied the narratives woven deeply into our patriarchal culture in ways that I did not even know about until much later in life. As a child growing up in the '80s and '90s, women were rarely the protagonists of the stories I read or watched. Heroes were nearly always male.

Where was the magic, mystery and power of women?

I have spent a lifetime foraging for it, re-membering, piece by piece, breath by breath, the lost story of my own womanhood: a story of relationship, breath, earth, animal, grief, joy, pleasure, blood, sex and sacrifice. I woke up, not to the prince, but to the fact that I had been duped. Duped by stories that did not serve me. In fact, the main stories of my culture had actually exploited my femininity and sold me a decorative and diminished version of what I was, and could be.

These stories encouraged me to overwork, override my needs and accommodate the patriarchal order of things that ignores the cyclical wisdom at the heart of a woman's body. This creates trauma in our bodies, disconnection from our natural rhythms, mutes our primal instincts and in my thirties left me washed up on the shore of my own life, feeling bereft and exhausted.

In order to reclaim what was lost, I entered the descent.

A descent is an initiation that challenges every notion we have of ourselves and our lives. Like an earthquake, it begins close in, at the epicentre of our sense of self and then ripples out, changing the landscape of our relationships, work, spirituality, core beliefs, sense of belonging and understanding of the world. It is an embodied feminine path of initiation, a process of death and rebirth. Similar to the physical birthing of a baby, the descent pulls us energetically downwards, drawing us out of our heads and back into the body and the Earth. It is a humbling rite of passage that delivers us, through to the depths of our embodied subconscious, to meet the seat of our own power and vulnerability. This powerful process often happens in the kitchen of our lives, uncelebrated, even unnoticed by others and sadly, as a result, is often undervalued. Our heroine's journeys are the stuff of our humanness, but are all too frequently shrouded in shame or passed off as a failure, rather than considered something to honour. This book is a call for that to change.

One who descends is one who is called beyond the known structures of the society in which they live.

The one who descends is foraging for another way.

These initiatory thresholds may arrive in many forms: the end of a relationship, a bereavement, coming out as gay, baby loss, baby longing, an abortion, illness, the loss of a role or money, birth and the journey into parenthood, or more recently, Covid. Whatever the catalyst, the descent is heralded by a significant shift in our lives that rocks the ground we thought we were standing on and brings us back down into the mud and sludge of our humanity, body and psychological shadow. Just as the caterpillar enters the cocoon to dissolve, so too does the heroine experience a sort of dissolution of her known self, through which she enters the process of transformation. In this way, the heroine's journey provides a map of human metamorphosis: a process of liquification, that takes us beyond what we think we can endure and delivers us into deeper intimacy with who we are and have always been.

The story of Inanna is the oldest known telling of the heroine's journey to the underworld and is over four thousand years old. Written by the woman who is said to be the world's first known poet, Enheduanna, it is a tale of harrowing loss, grief, surrender and rebirth.

I first discovered the myth by chance in Linda Hartley's book, *Servants of the Sacred Dream*. When I read it, all the lights switched on inside me. It was like lighting the corridors of a map that I had been navigating, but had not fully integrated or understood. Through this experience, I felt first-hand the vital importance of myth, for consecrating the heroine's journeys we undertake. Many of our cultural narratives and pursuits are based on how productive we are, what we can gain and how we can improve our shiny human exteriors. The heroine's journey does the opposite: it asks us to remove our masks, shed our skin and arrive humble and naked in the underworld of our being.

Though the heroine's journey does still exist within our culture, and certainly our lives, we do not always give credence to these initiatory processes, or adequately recognise them as the heroic journeys that they are. I think this is in part because heroism is traditionally associated with will, valour and capability, rather than courage to surrender. Culturally, surrender is not valued but is instead equated with weakness. Additionally, we don't feel like a heroine when we are in the midst of the descent – it feels more like breaking down.

The journey to the underworld happens slowly over time, and initially we may not consciously know we are in the descent. We could be mistaken for thinking that we are simply stuck in a series of very difficult changes that have no common thread. But though there may seem to be no coherence in what is unfolding, this is a sacred path and there are landmarks that we can learn to recognise along the way. Inanna's story provides a mythopoetic map for the journey that leads us towards humility, empathy, relationship and, ultimately, Love.

In the past, or in other cultures, there may have been an elder, shaman or holy person who would help us to see the deeper process at play and support us in the depths, and as we rise. But in an increasingly secular, mechanistic world, we are largely estranged from the culture of eldership. Our medical structures tend to pertain to the rational and scientific, at the exclusion of spirit and soul. On the whole, even psychotherapy has a tendency to sit closer to the medical than the spiritual. In terms of religion, the ceremonies of our monotheistic western father-based religions often do not provide holding for the more feminine embodied experience of spirituality that we experience in the heroine's journey. As author Estella Lauter observes, "In the myth of the crucifixion, the soul is attained in the sacrifice of the body and the identification with the Father." Conversely, the feminine path of spirituality requires that we re-enter the body, fully and wholly in all its complexity, as a divine expression of the Mother Earth and an alive expression of soul.

In modern times, many things feminine are still grossly undervalued. The story of descent and rising is no exception. Therefore, the heroine's journey is less known and less told than other myths. I feel this is not only a loss to the individual, it is a loss to us all. A culture that cannot descend is a culture that is not rooted in the Earth. The exile and suppression of the feminine inside of ourselves is directly reflected in our external abuse and disconnection from the Earth. It has tangible and drastic consequences. We are living in a time of mass extinction: species of plants, insects and animals are being lost daily. I believe we are experiencing collective trauma arising from the erosion of our deep ecology and loss of connection with our natural rhythms and each other.

Covid disrupted our habitual patterns and temporarily suspended our ability to continue on as we were. This has been highly challenging for many people, some of whom have lost jobs, identities, people they love and social contact. We are all being called to descend into the shadows that brought us here. It is complex, frightening and, at times, overwhelming. My feeling is that we need the old stories to help us traverse this unknown territory. Collectively and individually we are being asked to meet the heroine within.

This book is an exploration of the somatic lived experience of an ancient story. I learned about the Inanna-Ereshkigal myth first by living it. My writing is informed by my own heroine's journey and through the many people, mainly women, who I have worked with as a psychotherapist, a psychosexual somatic therapist, a women's initiatory guide, yoga teacher and breathworker. My work is dedicated to beholding people as they traverse these rites of passage and I have spent many years holding women's sacred circles working with the Inanna-Ereshkigal myth. I feel the primordial energies mapped through the characters alive in me, in my body and my relationships and I can hear and feel them reflected in the stories of others. My hope is to help more people access the myth's wisdom and depths.

Over the course of writing this book, I spoke to many women from different socioeconomic and cultural backgrounds about their personal experiences of the heroine's journey, in order to gather a range of stories that might speak to you. I want to acknowledge that I have heard many women of colour name that they still do not feel visible in a white dominated landscape. As a woman holding white privilege, it is important to me that I do something demonstrative in my work to address that.

A common theme for those who shared their stories with me was a feeling of utter aloneness: the belief that no one could possibly comprehend what was happening to them. This makes sense, as the descent is so all-consuming that, for a time, we lose the capacity to see very far outside what is happening to us. But, as personal as it feels, it is not only your story, though its unique shape is yours: the heroine's journey is a well-worn and vital path that may be experienced once, or at several times over the course of a life. It is universal. It cannot be avoided, though we try with all our might. It is not a sign of weakness or failure, nor of our exceptionality, but rather an essential process of stripping away what we have outgrown, of accepting all that we cannot resolve and composting outdated and stifling ideals. Rising can feel incomprehensible when we are so far down into the dark. It has to be this way, to teach us that we cannot control everything and that, at times, we must submit to the greater forces at work. So that when we do eventually rise, we do so with true compassion and our feet firmly rooted in the ground.

The heroine's journey does not just happen in our heads, it is a somatic experience that moves through all layers of our being. You are a living, walking, breathing mythology, so I invite you to experience this book in an embodied way. To support you I include enquiries and practices that you can work through as you read. I encourage you to devote some time to journalling, moving and emoting when you need to. The exercises I offer are there to help guide you, but by all means be creative with them and follow your own instinctual flow.

How can you embrace this book as a sacred practice?

I am not telling a new story. I am telling an ancient story that I believe has not been recognised enough. I write my reflections on it in the hope that it will encourage more people to retrieve its rites of passage into our impoverished secular landscape. We are parched and these teachings water the cracked earth of our soul life, slowing us down and tethering us to a deeper knowing and respect for the Earth, ourselves and those around us. A place where desperation can be transformed into faith, and faith into a loving purpose. This book is a retelling of an old myth, a myth that I believe holds medicine for our times.

A note to readers

This book explores much territory that we tend to travel in the dark, unspoken. There are many first-hand accounts of traumatic experiences in this book which some readers might find triggering. In modern times, there seems to be a tendency to think that we should not ever be triggered – that it is a 'bad thing'. But in reality we can never be completely safe from things that will activate or upset us. The heroine's journey by nature brings us closer to past wounding. Therefore, it is very likely that we will be triggered as we descend. Though very uncomfortable and sometimes distressing, being triggered can in fact be a sign, a call from the Ereshkigal within us, for help and support.

As you read, I invite you to slow down enough to keep checking in with your body and emotions. One way we tend to deal with being triggered is to rush over material and override the feelings that are arising inside of us, or panic and enter our flight/fight response. If this happens, I suggest that you pause, put the book down and pay conscious attention to what is here. Notice your breathing, any physical tensions, numbness or lots of sensations, thoughts becoming scrambled or feeling blank – all these can be signs of overwhelm, and this list is not exhaustive.

If difficult feelings come up please do take time to journal, rest, digest and try to be kind to yourself. And, if needed, I recommend that you seek out a therapist or trusted person in your life for help and support.

A note on language

My main focus in this book is women and women's stories. Since the vast majority of my work and experience has been centred around the embodied experiences of women who were born female and identify as women, the language and content of this book reflects this. Though of course, men and gender-diverse people may be called to descend as well.

The terms masculine and feminine have become viewed as problematic by some because they are associated with confining gender norms. Therefore, it is important to emphasise that when I speak about feminine and masculine I am not talking about gender. I am referring to the creative energies of *eros*, that animate us and make us want to make love to our lives and each other. Regardless of sex or gender, what do we associate with these energies and how do they move in us? How do we relate to them personally and collectively? These questions are a part of the journey.

Chapter 1
THE HEROINE'S JOURNEY

From the Great Above, we opened our ears to the Great Below.

Sivani Mata is burgeoning on adolescence and is in the fragile transition from girl to woman, when first her grandma dies, then her godmother – who was her most trusted adult in the world – and then her father. She has just started to bleed and, at the threshold of womanhood, the supports that held her disappear. She cannot grieve, she spins off into teenagehood alone. She starts to descend.

Sophie has always wanted to be a mother, it was never a question. Now in her thirties she has been trying for over two years and is realising that it may not happen for her. She has been living her menstrual wisdom for years, she has been doing 'all the right things' but still nothing is happening. She starts to descend.

The descent starts with a moan, a call from deep inside, almost impossible to hear in the noise of daily life, but ever-present. Under the polished surface of existence there is something dark knocking at the door.

The Goddess Inanna is Queen of the Upperworld, she has power, respect and a good life. On the outside, everything seems fine, but there is something inside calling for her, something unmet, unknown, but also undeniable.

Her sister Ereshkigal is in exile, she has been 'down there' for years. It's one of those family issues that no one talks about. It's not been talked about for so long that it seems normal. But Inanna finds it unsettling: surely it's not normal? It's all she has ever known, so she isn't sure, but she is tired of the silence. More there for not being there, she sees Ereshkigal in her dreams and feels her absence.

Rejected by her family and upperworld society, Ereshkigal became Queen of the Underworld. She is the one that the upperworld will not admit, the one who gets blamed and shamed, the one who we ostracise and who the media burn at the modern witches' stake. She is the one we are encouraged to forget: life is busy and she is not a priority. She who it is too painful to acknowledge, or who has simply been buried through the years of overcoming.

In this split, Inanna has lost her sister, and both of them are in pain. The estrangement appears as this unexplained feeling inside: a moan, a howl, something unexpressed. Inanna hasn't exactly got the language for it, maybe it's beyond words. Despite this, she knows she has to follow the call.

But the underworld is forbidden to upperworld people: they do not look below. If you want to stay in favour, you don't go down there because it never ends well. The Sky Gods forbid it. For Inanna to descend, she must go against many social conventions and risk her life as she knows it.

In Inanna's wisdom she calls to her handmaiden, Ninshubur, to be her witness and watch for her return. In our own lives this might be a therapist or a close friend. It's also the part of us that can watch for us, our inner witness. Before she goes, Inanna instructs Ninshubur,

"If I am not back in seven days bang the drum for me. Call for help. Help me return."

In preparation for the descent, Inanna gathers the *me:*[*] her crown, lapis beads, necklaces, breastplate, gold bracelets, measuring rod and robe. She arrives at the gates of the underworld and tells the Gatekeeper she wants to enter. When Ereshkigal hears Inanna's intention to descend she is enraged. Ereshkigal is the neglected sister, the dark side of the feminine, the ravenous, furious, rejected, unloved, lonely, exiled one. How dare she who is all light think that she can come to visit

---

[*]   Powerful upperworld objects.

the *kur?** She demands that Inanna must come naked and bowed low.

Inanna must pass through seven gates to descend. At each gate, an aspect of Inanna's upperworld identity is taken from her, in a ruthless process of stripping her bare. Through this she loses her old identities and sense of belonging in the upperworld. This is the way we re-enter the body, how we reconnect with what has been hidden in the flesh of our existence. This is the path of surrender.

At the first gate her crown is taken from her. Inanna exclaims,

"What is this?"

The Gatekeeper replies,

"Quiet, Inanna, the ways of the underworld are perfect, they may not be questioned." [1†]

It makes absolutely no sense to her: she is queen and that is her crown, how dare they take it away? In the upperworld, it's all about what we can accumulate, what we take on, what we achieve. But in the underworld, this holds no significance. All upperworld objects will be relinquished when we enter the *kur*. We all die naked, nothing can be taken with us.

At the second gate her lapis beads are removed and again she says,

"What is this?"

And the same reply comes,

"Quiet, Inanna, the ways of the underworld are perfect, they may not be questioned."

At the third gate, her necklaces are removed from her breast and she continues to ask,

"What is this?"

She is told,

"Quiet, Inanna, the ways of the underworld are perfect, they may not be questioned."

At each gate, another one of her upperworld garments is removed. Another aspect of her identity has to be composted so that she can meet herself, her deeper ecology and her dark sister. The upperworld laws hold no currency in

---

* Another name for the underworld. It is said to mean 'the world of the dead' and also 'mountain'.

† My telling of the myth is based on the structure of the poem as translated by Diane Wolkstein and Samuel Kramer. The direct quotations from the poem are numbered see references for more.

the underworld, whose ruthless rites of passage take from us everything that is surplus to the journey. We cannot stay as we are, we must yield to a new rhythm, that pulsates beyond our current understanding and values. It makes no sense, and yet we go, putting one foot in front of the other into the dark.

At each threshold, Inanna descends deeper into her body and the body of the Earth. She enters the dark to come closer to everything within herself that she has not yet consciously known. At the final gate, her robes are removed and though she knows the answer, the last vestige of hope and fight compels her to ask once more,

"What is this?"

And still the reply is the same,

"The laws of the underworld are perfect Inanna, they may not be questioned."

The crown lying on the floor, the measuring stick, her robes…have been taken, along with all the old stories about what she was and how she should be. All that was expected of her and all that was not allowed. It is all dissolving. She crosses the seventh gate naked, completely stripped bare. As she stands in the underworld, tired, cold and disorientated, she lifts her head and sees her sister Ereshkigal. She steps towards her, but Ereshkigal is not up for a loving sisterly reunion. She shows Inanna no mercy. All her rage roars upwards, she strikes Inanna and impales her on a meat hook and leaves her to rot. There, Inanna enters full submission, as her upperworld identity dies.

Inanna hangs there as a corpse for three days and three nights.

Meanwhile, above ground, in the upperworld, Inanna's handmaiden Ninshubur is getting increasingly worried. She has been waiting for Inanna and has set up a lament for her. She bangs the drum in the assembly places, she offers up her prayers, but when Inanna still does not appear she dresses herself in a sack cloth, and sets out to visit the temples of the Sky Gods to appeal for help. This is what grief does, it leaves us empty as a beggar and bereft to the core.

First she visits Father Enlil and appeals for his help,

"Father Enlil, Inanna has not returned from the underworld
You must help.
Please do not let your daughter be lost."

But Father Enlil replies in anger and distaste,

"My daughter craved the Great Below.
I no longer know her.

She who goes to the underworld does not return,
She should have known better.
I have nothing more to say."

Father Enlil is a typical Sky God. As far as he is concerned, Inanna has fallen from grace and upset the hierarchy, which must be upheld at all costs. Inanna is not the daughter he thought she was. His rigid beliefs prevent any empathy or compassion to arise for Inanna. She made the decision to descend and now she must suffer the consequences.

Ninshubur's loyalty is unswerving, she will not be dissuaded, so she tries Father Nanna. But he gives the same response,

"Inanna should not have entered the underworld.
It is no place for a woman like her.
She had temples, she had a good husband and a good life.
She must have lost her mind.
I have nothing more to say."

These are the men who have ruled the kingdom. They enjoy their privileges and benefit from the structures that they believe keep order in the upperworld. They will not unthrone themselves willingly. Their only interest is keeping things balanced in their favour and they are willing to sacrifice their daughter to maintain that, if that is what is required. The Sky Gods are the part of us that stays safe in our heads: the rational, the superior, the judge and the jury. They are the ones in us that do not want to admit our humanness and who refuse to feel. They cannot empathise, they will not be humbled and they will not help.

> *Ninshubur soon begins to realise that she is*
> *knocking on the door of the wrong Gods.*

But she is unsure who else she can ask, so she travels to the temple of Enki, the God of the Seas, in the hope that he will be willing to help. When she tells him of Inanna's plight, he immediately wants to help. Enki is creative and empathic, he is a gardener and a soulful Sky God, who has been initiated into the dark feminine himself. He pulls the earth out from under his fingernails and fashions the dirt into two little creatures: a *galatur* and a *kugarra*, creatures that are neither male nor female. He tells them,

"Go to the underworld,

Enter the door like flies.
Ereshkigal, the Queen of the Underworld is about to give birth...
When she cries, 'Oh! Oh! My inside!'
Cry also, 'Oh! Oh! My inside!'
When she cries, 'Oh! Oh! My outside!'
Cry also, 'Oh! Oh! My outside!'
The queen will be pleased.
She will offer you a gift.
Ask her only for the corpse that hangs from the hook on the wall.
One of you will sprinkle the food of life on it.
The other will sprinkle the water of life.
Inanna will arise." [2]

The *galatur* and *kugarra* are small as flies and can go through the gates of the underworld undetected by the gatekeeper. They go in search of Ereshkigal and manage to find her. Just as Enki said, she is making birthing sounds,

Ereshkigal moans,

"Oh! Oh! My belly!"

They moan,

"Oh! Oh! Your belly!"

She groans,

"Oh! Oh! My back!"

They groan,

"Oh! Oh! My back!"

As she sighs,

"Ah! Ah! My heart!"

They sigh,

"Ah! Ah! Your heart!"

After a time, she looks up at them and asks,

"Who are you,
Moaning-groaning-sighing with me?
If you are gods, I will bless you
If you are mortals, I will give you a gift
I will give you the water-gift, the river in its fullness.
I will give you the grain-gift, the fields in harvest." [3]

Ereshkigal has been alone for so long, moaning into the cavernous space of the underworld with only her own voice as an echo. These creatures are her mid-wives and they bring empathy as their gift. She is so moved by them, that she offers them the gift of food, nourishment to bring back life, and water, to help the river of life flow again. This symbolises the new life that can move when somebody sits with us in our pain and can actually hear what we are going through.

They ask for Inanna's corpse and she grants them their request. But as Inanna is about to ascend, the judges of the underworld seize her. They decree that no one leaves the underworld unmarked and they demand a sacrifice. If Inanna is to return to the upperworld, she must send another to the underworld in her place. They send the *galla*, demons of the underworld, who flank Inanna as she returns. If she does not make a sacrifice she will be haunted by her demons. These demons symbolise the parts of us that are not yet fully integrated. They want what they want at any cost. If we do not make a sacrifice, then our journey will be aborted and we will be held in purgatory. If we don't give them the sacrifice they need, the demons will stand like a fence between us and our lives.

If Inanna wants to be fully alive, she must now learn the lesson
that she cannot have everything – she must make a sacrifice.

As she returns to the upperworld, the first person she meets is Ninshubur, who is dressed in a soiled sackcloth. Ninshubur is so delighted to see Inanna that she throws herself at her feet in relief and joy. In this gesture she embodies the humility and loyalty of the witness that is so vital for our journey.

As the *galla* go to seize Ninshubur, Inanna stops them,

"No! Ninshubur, is my constant support.
She is my sukkal who gives me wise advice.
She is my warrior who fights by my side.
Because of her my life was saved.
I will never give Ninshubur to you." [4]

Inanna recognises the importance of Ninshubur and tells the demons, *"no"*. Her voice was taken in the descent, but as she rises she reclaims it – her words are assertive and clear.

As she continues on her journey, she meets her two sons. Also dressed in soiled sack cloths, they too have been grieving the loss of their mother. They throw themselves at the feet of Inanna. As the demons go to take them she again says,

"No, I will never give my sons to you".

When she finally arrives at her city, there, by the big apple tree, she finds her husband Dumuzi, the King. Dumuzi is dressed in shining robes, lounging casually on Inanna's throne. In her absence, he has usurped her. He does not rise to greet Inanna. He shows no humility, only arrogance. It is for this reason that she knows instantly: he is the one who must be sacrificed. He is the masculine inside us who cannot admit his grief, who is unwilling to change. He is lost in a sense of his own splendour and fears the dark feminine. He does not have the capacity to acknowledge Inanna's descent. Though he is her husband and she loves him, Inanna knows that he is the one that she must sacrifice. He too must be initiated into the ways of the underworld. The King must die.

But Dumuzi will not go willingly. He does not want to look at his shadow and he will do anything to avoid his fate. He turns into a snake to slither away into hiding. He is the part of us, or others, who is afraid of transformation and clings to the safety of sameness.

Dumuzi hides, but the demons are relentless and follow him from one hiding place to the next: they will not leave without a sacrifice. In his despair, Dumuzi calls to his sister, Geshtinanna for help. Geshtinanna is the embodiment of compassion. She is grief-stricken for her brother and is deeply concerned for his plight. She appeals to Inanna for mercy on Dumuzi's behalf and offers to sacrifice herself in his place. Inanna is so moved by Geshtinanna's love for her brother that it softens her to her own grief for her husband. Inanna must now stand in her agency with compassion. To do so is to embody a different kind of authority.

Together Geshtinanna and Inanna find Dumuzi weeping, all his grandeur has dissolved. Inanna takes him by the hand and tells him that though he will still have to go to the underworld, he will only go for half the year, and on his return, Geshtinanna will take his place for the other half of the year. Despite any personal feelings she may have, she has learned from Ereshkigal the hard way, that the laws of the underworld must not be questioned. She makes the sacrifice not out of vengeance or to punish, but with compassion and consciousness. From this wisdom, she becomes an initiatress into the feminine mysteries.

Inanna places Dumuzi in the hands of the eternal. [5]

And so, the cycle is complete. The masculine, in the form of Dumuzi, and the feminine, in the form of Geshtinanna, have entered a new partnership.

Geshtinanna is vital for the completion of the cycle, because through her we find our compassion. Compassion that gives us the capacity to be with both our own suffering and the suffering of others, with loving kindness. Compassion to fully admit what needs to be admitted, even though it may hurt us to do so. Compassion that gives us the courage to descend not once, but again and again, as many times as we need to keep learning and living life. With compassion and gratitude life can flow, even in the most difficult of circumstances. This is an initiation of death and rebirth, that requires all of our courage, humility and endurance.

The underworld is calling. Will you enter?

Chapter 2
ENTERING THE DARK

You darkness that I come from
I love you more than all the fires that fence in the world
For the fire makes a circle of light for everyone,
and then no one outside learns of you.
But the dark pulls in everything:
Shapes and fires, animals and myself,
How easily it gathers them;
Powers and people —
And I feel a great presence might be moving beside me,
I have faith in nights.

Rainer Maria Rilke, translated by Robert Bly

When I descended, I learned there was another story of my life. Not the one that I knew, but the under-story that had been playing beneath what I thought I knew about who I was. In this under-story lived the shadow stream, the current that pulled the waves on the surface of my life: wounding, desire, rage, longing, vitality, strength and the roots of my misguided ideas and ideals lived there. The heroine's path I walked to my own underworld was led by love and desire, but it landed me in grief, complexity and painful awakening: an awakening that I am utterly grateful for. What I was subconsciously searching for was the red thread of my feminine lineage, but it was buried and entangled. Only through digging in the dark could it be uncovered. I was looking for another way, and through this search, I became the unwitting heroine of my own mythology.

I was Inanna, and the one I was unknowingly
searching for was my sister, Ereshkigal.

When Inanna descends, she makes a choice to enter the dark. When we see in the dark, we do not look through the cones of our eyes as we do in the light. Instead, the light that's available is received by the rods in our eyes, meaning that we see less colour and look more peripherally – we have to widen our view. This also heightens our other senses and brings us into our bodies.

The descent is also a process of arriving in the body and, through that, the depths of the underworld. Coming from a society that praises the rational, visible and quantifiable, we may not immediately trust the dark or easily adapt to this new landscape. I wonder if this is one of the reasons why the heroine's journey is less written about, as it is less seen, but also difficult to capture without losing the essential essence of what we are trying to describe. To widen our view, our pupils literally become more open. This opening and widening to the dark heightens our sensitivity and awareness. In the light of day, we are bombarded by colour, information and noise; night is quieter, more mysterious, and demands a visceral expansion of our awareness to navigate. The other time our eyes dilate this way is when we see someone we are attracted to: our pupils widen to take in more of them. We so often associate the dark with fear, but actually the dark is the thing that literally opens us to love and enables us to be receptive to the world of our longing. We were created in the dark womb of our mother; our first music was the heartbeat and our first home was the dark.

Without loving relationships, humans fail to flourish, even if all of their basic needs are met. 'Love lost' is one of the most powerful forms of stress and trauma. We now understand that the causes and consequences of love or its absence are grounded in a biology that operates largely below the level of human consciousness.

Dr Sue Carter, *The Biology of Love*

This place *below human consciousness* is the underworld of our being and the place that the heroine must enter. Whilst the hero puts on armour and goes out into the world for his journey, the heroine takes her armour off as she descends into her body, unprocessed trauma and life. The heroine's journey offers a spiritual path that does not ask us to deny any aspect of our experience, or who we are. Rather than building up, we are asked to come back down to Earth, as we meet and embrace all parts of ourselves. The hero pursues self-preservation, whilst the heroine dismantles the self she has known in order to discover what she is underneath. When I spoke with yoga teacher Angela Farmer, who has worked with the Inanna-Ereshkigal myth for decades, she told me that,

"The Sumerian myth of Inanna appeared towards the end of the astrological Taurian period and Taurus is the great representative of Mother Goddess. Something was changing, just as now, the Piscean age, with all its systems and religions is cracking and dispersing for a new Aquarian age to emerge. In that time, the Goddess was no longer respected and women were dis-empowered. Inanna the great and beloved Goddess had been put up in the sky. Women were split apart, their wholeness replaced by the extremes of 'exotic superstar, sex idol' and the old hag or ugly witch that features so much in our Northern myths, who was down in the underworld. I think this has been felt tremendously. If a woman feels ashamed of her body, is abused, hurt or denied privileges, a split may occur in what she presents to the outer world and what is hidden or buried inside her. Then, like Inanna, she holds a deep yearning for truth and wholeness. The myth's courageous 'inner' journey shows us the way to reclaim ourselves, heal and recover our loss."

Now, as our times are shifting, many old paradigms so deeply ingrained into our structures, institutions and psyches are being outed and challenged. Ereshkigal's moan is getting louder: she wants to be heard, included and seen. The heroine's journey is a quest to re-member, reclaim and reconnect with our exiled feminine. If we are to arrive in wholeness, then we must be willing embrace Ereshkigal as a part of Inanna. We have to embrace our shadow, including those aspects of ourselves that we may deem as failures, weaknesses or too painful, as a valuable part of who we are.

The Feminine Vision Quest

In a male-centric world, initiations are often sold as something we go and *do*, whereas the path of feminine initiation arrives through being – it is primarily an inward, rather than an external quest. The material for it is happening right here, whilst we navigate work, relationships, or the school run. The heroine's journey is initiated by what's happening in the stuff of your life, in the emotional and visceral landscapes of your being.

> *Women find their way back to themselves not by moving up and out into the light like men, but by moving down into the depths of the ground of their being. [...] The spiritual experience for women is one of moving more deeply into self rather than out of self.*
>
> **Maureen Murdock, *The Heroine's Journey***

I can sense some feminists raging at this idea, but stay with me. What if the notion that we have to go out to *do* our initiations is the same patriarchal narrative that tells us we have to *do* our lives in a particular way to be of value? I am not saying that women must only stay at home to vision quest, whilst men go out on grand adventures. I have plenty of female friends who have chosen to do vision quests out in the wild, and more power to them. But, my curiosity is: why is it that the outward journey is sold as desirable, whilst the actual stuff of our lives and the inward journey are so undervalued? The heroine's journey is the other path, the one right under our noses. The stuff of daily life is rife with grace: births, deaths, raising children or not, heartbreaks, relationship difficulties, work...all of this is part of, not separate from, the sacred. But it doesn't sell as well as the grand quest or gesture. The hero's journey is a valuable rite of passage, but the heroine's journey is of equal value. Yet it has not been equally valued. Now is as good a time as any to change that.

Traditionally, the female vision quest happens through our life experiences and through the descent into menstruation (also known as moontime). The menstrual cycle is a microcosm of the descent and rising. Resting, dreaming and yielding to our moontime is one way of contacting the underworld within. The womb is a woman's embodied underworld and the descending energy of the bleed is the death part of the cycle, where we can shed what is ready to be released and rebirth ourselves anew into the coming cycle.

Sadly, the dominant stories of Western culture venerate masculine energy which dominates and is thought to be superior to all things feminine. The story that many women have swallowed whole is not that menstruation is our power, but that it is a shameful weakness. Therefore, an inherent part of the heroine's journey for many women is a remembering of our embodied cyclical wisdom. In my own descent, my relationship to both the moon and my bleed became life sustaining threads that I followed. In our cultural paradigms, we command and dominate our bodies. We shape, tone, snip, shave and coerce them into a palatable, socially acceptable shape: a shape that can survive in a man's world. The popular stories of our Western culture praise this paradigm, as Lara Owen author of *Her Blood is Gold*, illuminates,

For the past few thousand years, certainly in Judeo-Christian culture (and many others) being female is seen as a Bad Thing. We have had a lineage of descent that honours the male over the female, and a preference for giving birth to sons. Consequently, that which is special to the female has tended to be denigrated, whereas that which pertains to the male has been prized and respected.

Menstruation has even been thought to be a curse given to women to bear for the sin of Eve. Eve who was cast out of the garden of Eden, just as Ereshkigal was cast out of the upperworld. These stories, so deeply embedded into our religions, culture and bodies, have led to the shaming and suppression of our blood wisdom. A shame that for many women, sits at the foundation of our womanhood and relationship with the feminine.

If we are to fully embrace Ereshkigal, we must also embrace our own wild bodies, in all their beauty, strength, mess and fragility.

Rewilding Through the Descent

Our descents always seem to have a catalyst, something that compels us to descend. Illness, injury and incapacitation can be a catalyst that takes us back into the wild landscape of the body. I spoke to Claire Patrick, about her experience of the descent,

"I had a really big job in TV in a popular medical documentary series that uses hospital scenarios to tell people's stories. It was a wonderful thing to be part of, but you are exposed to extreme amounts of trauma day-to-day, and I was putting myself under an immense amount of pressure in that role. My lack of boundaries, my lack of self-care, my subjugation of what I needed over what I thought everyone else required, all came to a head. Throughout this process of taking myself to the brink with my work, I was having extreme headaches, but I couldn't bear to take time off to go to the GP. It was only when I finished that job that I went to the doctor and they sent me for a scan. Before I knew it, I was in A&E myself, because they discovered a very large cyst in my brain. I went in for surgery that was supposed to be relatively benign, because it was just exploratory brain surgery, but it caused a haemorrhage and I was extremely, extremely ill. It was really terrifying, because I was in this place that I had seen in making my documentaries, where something terrible happens and nothing scientific can tell you what the outcome is going to be. And you're held in this state of flux, where the only way through is extreme surrender and extreme acceptance."

What Claire describes is exactly where Inanna lands as she enters the underworld and asks the gatekeeper, *"What is this?"* to which he repeatedly replies, *"Quiet Inanna, the ways of the underworld are perfect, they may not be questioned."* What Claire met is the place where our human limits – of being able to fix and control outcomes – end. She continues,

"On the face of it, it was the worst thing that could possibly happen, and at the same time, there was an extreme awakening of sorts happening that was very powerful. The thing was, that if I was at risk of having a heart attack and they were able to say, 'If you do this and this and this, it might be alright,' I would have had a road map that was action-taking. But when your brain is bleeding and medically it's deemed as unsafe to intervene as it is to leave it, there is nothing to do. There was no one to turn to, nowhere to turn to, and there was nothing pro-active to be done and that was absolute."

Claire had to submit to the process, just as Inanna submits to the laws of the underworld. Though her experience is an extreme one, what Claire's haemorrhage led her to is the deeper listening that is required on the heroine's journey. I asked Claire more about what she leant on in that space of not knowing.

"Prior to that, for about five years, I had quite a deep spiritual practice of meditation and lots of inner work and I would book-end my day with meditation practices. But it was as if I had two chambers in my life, one was like, 'this is my zen, calm self' and then there was the, what felt like, life or death, of my career and my very head-led panicky, physiologically triggering work life. They existed in tandem and I didn't quite know how to reconcile the two: it didn't make sense to me."

One way to cope with life is to keep going at all costs. This is also one way that we keep Ereshkigal in exile – by being too busy to feel. The *life and death* charge that Claire refers to feeling shows up in the body as a strong sense of urgency to keep going, even when we are frazzled, ill or in need of a rest. This pattern is symptomatic of hyper-arousal in the nervous system.

The autonomic nervous system (ANS) plays an essential role in our emotional and physiological responses to stress and trauma. The ANS has two primary branches within it: the sympathetic nervous system that activates our fight and flight response and the parasympathetic nervous system that shifts us into rest and digest. Ideally, we naturally oscillate between activity and rest, sympathetic to parasympathetic to aid activity, healthy digestion, immune system function and sleep. But when we have experienced trauma or are stressed, we can get stuck in hyper- or hypo-arousal patterns. Hyper being over-active, meaning we may find it very difficult to down-regulate into rest and digest again. Or hypo-arousal, which is a kind of shut down in the system that can show up as feelings of lethargy, disconnection or numbness.

In my experience, the impulse underneath the hyper-active work patterns that Claire describes almost always originates from the wound that Ereshkigal is holding. Claire shared with me that in her familial lineage there was a history of poverty, illiteracy and alcohol abuse. A response to this kind of familial trauma can be a strong drive to be a success and work really hard. The compulsion of the wounding, combined with the societal pressures of living in a capitalist society, can make the need for success feel *like life and death* and at some point, it possibly was life or death. But the trauma pattern that continues to play can keep us trapped in survival mode for many years, not able to fully thrive because we can't surrender, we cannot stop. On the outside we may appear highly functional, but, as Claire names, underneath she was *subjugating her needs*. In order to subjugate our needs, we must exile Ereshkigal: we must not admit our wounded self. Illness is one way that this cycle can get interrupted, and when it does, it is both terrible and, as Claire describes, *one of the most liberating experiences of my life*.

In the poem 'Wild Geese' Mary Oliver famously says,

> *You do not have to be good.*
> *You do not have to walk on your knees*
> *for a hundred miles through the desert repenting.*
> *You only have to let the soft animal of your body,*
> *love what it loves.*

Time and again, I see these words melt the Inanna, the good daughter, the hard worker, the one striving for perfection, in the people I work with. Ereshkigal's moan is the moan of the *soft animal* of the body. She calls us back to the wild one inside. In her book, *Women Who Run with the Wolves*, Clarissa Pinkola Estés names,

> *Wildlife and the Wild Woman are both endangered species. Over time we*
> *have seen the feminine instinctive nature looted, driven back and overbuilt.*
> *For long periods it has been mismanaged like the wildlife and the wildlands.*
> *For several thousand years, as soon and as often as we turn our backs, it is*
> *relegated to the poorest land in the psyche. The spiritual lands of the Wild*
> *Woman have throughout history been plundered or burnt, dens bulldozed*
> *and natural cycles forced into unnatural rhythms to please others. [...] The*
> *modern woman is a blur of activity. She is pressured to be all things to all*
> *people. The old knowing is long overdue.*

Even our spiritual practices can become a part of the *blur of activity*, a way to keep it all under control. Will-based spiritual practices can actually feed the same nervous system loop as our other survival mechanisms. This might look healthy on the outside, but on the inside it may actually be contributing to the suppression of our own vulnerability. I experienced this in my own spiritual practice, which for years was a daily practice of yoga asana that I would do *no matter what*. The will-based discipline of this practice did yield something valuable, but it also had an unacknowledged shadow. For women living in such a masculine dominated society, I question, is a masculine, will-based spiritual practice what is truly needed? My own heroine's journey taught me the hard way, that though I was listening on one level, on another level I was bone tired and I had not admitted it. What I needed was surrender. Surrender can allow us to touch something that our will cannot access. As Claire so beautifully depicts,

> "During the worst moments of the brain issue, there was a serene lake inside me that I touched. And I had touched it, but not through efforting... What that's taught me as a place you're able to access as a human being, a place you're able to go, was completely life-changing."

Birth and death take us into another realm where normal life is suspended. Here we may perhaps touch upon something we have been too busy to feel: a sort of time outside of time, where everything that seems so big day-to-day is put into a new field of vision. As Claire says,

> "It's almost like the prescription of your glasses has changed. In fact, it's like everyone else is walking around without their glasses on. But the material realities and societal expectations are still there.
> You hear stories that end with, 'and then this happened and all was well,' but it's not like that. The wellness world sells you a version of what will happen if you follow your heart, but actually it's really messy and full of complexity."

The heroine's journey is a soul clear-out that will challenge even our most well-honed coping strategies and bring us into a deeper relationship with ourselves and beyond.

The Spirit of the Times and the Spirit of the Depths

In his *Red Book,* psychoanalyst and founder of analytical psychology Carl Jung, said that there were two layers of humanity: the spirit of the times and the spirit of the depths. The spirit of the times being the narratives and drives of the times in which we live, created by humans. The spirit of the depths being the soul that underpins our day-to-day existence in something greater and beyond human creation. In a sense, Inanna can be seen to represent the spirit of the times, and Ereshkigal the spirit of the depths. In our secular society, soul life has arguably been trampled on by the spirit of the times. Our technological age has changed our relationship to everything, and we are now bombarded by information at a speed that was never possible before. Never has the spirit of the times been at such an oppositional pace to the spirit of the depths, which has its own natural pace and will not be hurried.

How do we even contact soul in a world that is so avaricious?

Contrary to our culture that primes us to go out to seek fulfilment, Inanna descends inwards because on some level she knows it is an inevitable part of her journey to maturity. In choosing to descend, she chooses to risk her own significance and put down her upperworld identities to discover what she is beyond those ideals.

Collectively, if we open to the spirit of our depths, then we will have to undergo collective transformation. Unless the changing weather systems have already displaced you from your home, to an extent we can still see the climate crisis as something 'over there', whereas Covid made it personal. Many people lost jobs, identities, support systems and people they dearly love, awakening us to loss. Our losses are portals to the underworld. As Jung states,

The spirit of the depths forced me to speak to my soul, to call upon her as a living and self-existing being. I had to become aware that I had lost my soul. From this we learn how the spirit of the depths considers the soul: he sees her as a living and self-existing being, and with this he contradicts the spirit of this time for whom the soul is a thing dependent on man, which lets herself be judged and arranged, and whose circumference we can grasp. I had to accept that what I had previously called my soul was not at all my soul, but a dead system. Hence, I had to speak to my soul as to something far off and unknown, which did not exist through men but through whom I existed.

I feel the *living and existing being* to which Jung refers, is personified by the essential essence held inside of Ereshkigal. Inside of our shadow and suffering is essential life energy, not only *our* personal life energy, but that which enlivens and connects all things. In other words, our divinity is not separate from, but inextricably linked to our human mess. One way to realise this is by entering the dark of the depths and remembering that we are part of a much bigger web than we can possibly comprehend with our minds. The heroine's journey humbles us enough to acknowledge our individual, structural and collective wounding. It pulls our human wounded self and our divine spiritual and soulful self together. It provides an ancient map that guides us home.

Chapter 3

UNDERSTORY –
THE INANNA-ERESHKIGAL
MYTH AS AN ANCIENT MAP
OF TRAUMA INTEGRATION

It is astonishing to me that Inanna's journey essentially tells the story of trauma integration. In the spirit of our times, science is often our default go-to for information, but the wisdom held in mythological maps has a lot to teach us.

It is the weaving together of heroic myth and biology ('mytho-biology') that will help us comprehend the roots and mysterium tremendum of trauma.

Peter Levine, *In an Unspoken Voice*

The myth of Inanna's descent originated over 4000 years ago in ancient Sumer – now modern-day Iraq – long before the kind of research and modern scientific knowledge we have about trauma today. And yet, it describes the process amazingly well. Inanna goes to the dark of her embodied subconscious to tend to her wounds and free the life energy trapped there. This is exactly what we do when we titrate and work with trauma. The root of the word 'trauma' is from Greek and means 'wound'. Whatever the catalyst for our descents in adult life, what we get called towards is an old wound, the parts of us that have been exiled and needing our attention, perhaps for a lifetime.

Inanna is the upperworld part of us, the part that we identify and recognise as our self. This includes our work, our ways of communicating, our known ways of coping with life, being in relationships and getting love. Inanna is our conscious self and possibly our 'successful' self, the parts that we are willing to show. But Ereshkigal, our exiled self, is always there. She might manifest as the depression that routinely comes to visit, or the freeze we experience when we have sex, or the rage we feel, or the stuck feeling in our throat when we want to cry, or speak and can't. Entombed inside the dark pain of all these responses is pure, vital, life energy. Ereshkigal is the Dark Goddess and the personification of our wounded and soulful self. How can she be both, when the soul is so often painted as this beautiful untouched thing? Here we encounter one of the many paradoxes held in the tapestry of the heroine's journey: one of the ways that we can touch what is untouchable and unbreakable, is through our brokenness. Therefore, our personal human story is a portal that takes us beyond what we know, into contact with what is impersonal and vast. If we can withstand the heroine's journey, we may find that within our worst fears, and most difficult feelings, lie some of our greatest gifts. As renowned trauma therapist, Gabor Maté describes,

> *Metaphorically, if a wound is raw it's very sensitive, so when you touch it, it really hurts. Trauma induces these sensitive spots, that when touched later in life, cause a big pain reaction. On the other hand, wounds cause scar tissue, which doesn't have any nerve endings. So as wounds heal, they're not flexible, the tissue is rigid and can't grow. So, on the one hand the wound is sensitive and on the other hand it's rigid. You can't grow emotionally or spiritually, it's constrictive.*

The catalysts for our descents are the events, relationships and experiences that touch this *raw spot* in us. Something happens that propels us towards the root of an earlier wounding, often from childhood, and there we encounter all that has been hiding within us – all of our unprocessed feelings and suffering. It's like when you pull a piece of treasure out of the sea and attached to it are years of netting, rubbish, some dead sea life, and all sorts of build-up. Our wounds are like this. Grief for one thing tends to dredge up all the other griefs and unmet parts of ourselves that have been waiting for our attention.

Meeting Our Unmet Wounds

I spoke to Trista Hendren, founder of Girl God Books, about her heroine's journey,

> "I basically lost absolutely everything, except my children, who I could have lost. I was threatened with losing them. Their father came from a lot of money, and he was threatening me with losing custody over parental alienation. Basically, they discredited it, but it still gets used all the time against women in family courts all over the world. When I decided I would leave him, because he had drug and alcohol issues and was very emotionally and financially abusive, he and his family were like, 'You're going to pay.' So I ended up losing my house, I was bankrupt, I lost absolutely everything.
>
> About the same time, over four years, I think I counted that I lost over seventeen people in my life, including my three remaining grandparents. I cared for all of them, prior to their deaths. My children were very young and I was going through this very difficult relationship with my ex. And in the same period, there was a financial crash, so no one was buying houses. One of the worst moments was when I had to go and file for bankruptcy. I had spent thirteen years as a mortgage broker…and to be in that position myself was one of the lowest moments of my entire life. I remember just sitting with the attorney outside after and just sobbing. I could not stop sobbing for so long. That was the moment when I knew I had really lost everything."

Trista's story illustrates so well the way that the descent ricochets through our lives, affecting our work, family relationships, friendships, relationship to money, sexuality, our emotions, our whole sense of self. Trista was utterly stripped, like Inanna in the underworld, and this vulnerability led her back to her old wounds. Trista had been raised in the Church, and in our conversation she named how she was always "forced to be this good little girl, very quiet". But as she descended, she unearthed her rage,

"I always think of Alice Walker's quote, 'Healing begins where the wound was made' and I think these wounds are mostly from childhood. I was very much hurting and angry with my ex-husband, but also at the men in my family. I was molested by my step-father. My dad was a very good man, but he was very patriarchal and I don't think he understands what it is to be a woman, which I think is getting better now he is a bit older and retired. But I had to really actively try to come to terms with all that. For a long time, I pushed as far away as I could and I went very extreme. I don't want to say anti-man, but kind of anti-man. I went to place that for me now, is too far. I have a wonderful husband now and I have a wonderful son and male friends and other wonderful men in my life and I have come back into balance with the masculine. But back then, I was very angry."

The parts that were not nurtured in childhood are often the parts that we have exiled. But to live with parts of ourselves in exile impacts us deeply on a physical level. Because these experiences cannot be fully amputated, they live on inside the body. They are in our somatic experience and whether we realise it or not, the energy of them is playing out in our lives now, in who and what we are attracted to, our addictions and coping mechanisms and the ways we experience ourselves in the world. But we are often so busy living life, that we do not fully join the dots and even if we do, we can feel trapped, ashamed and powerless to change our patterns. The heroine is asked to admit and, importantly, feel the patterns.

When Inanna descends to meet Ereshkigal she enters a healing journey to embrace what she has abandoned inside of herself.

Capital T and Lower Case t Trauma

When we say trauma, we often think of big shocking events such as rape, war, a life-threatening accident, and these are of course, traumatic. We can call these capital T Traumas. But we also experience what can be referred to as lowercase t traumas. These small t traumas can be anything that happened too fast and too soon for us, or any experience that we were powerless or too overwhelmed to process. For example, having a cervical screening at the doctors and not having agency over the speculum being inserted, boundary violations, bullying, being shamed or shown up, religious trauma or verbal abuse and this list is far from exhaustive. In reality, trauma is a spectrum. Babette Rothschild and Bessel Van Der Kolk suggest that we take trauma seriously by not claiming it's there when it is not. So I want to recognise that acute capital T Trauma and Post Traumatic Stress Disorder (PTSD) can literally inhibit your ability to live your life and should not be confused with other suffering. But I also believe that we all have unprocessed material in our bodies that affects how we deal with life and the way that we relate. In short, trauma is a part of being human.

Fortunately, the ability to heal is also an inherent part of being human. One of the beautiful things about the Inanna-Ereshkigal myth is that it maps the heroine's descent down into our wounding *and* the ascent and integration back into life-fullness. I believe that it is our innate drive towards healing that compels Inanna to descend and rise again. We have all had experiences that hurt us, that were too much to process at the time. Ereshkigal remembers all of these experiences and holds them down in the underworld of the body with her, in what are referred to as our *implicit memories*. These are memories that may not be consciously remembered in the mind, but are held in the body and importantly in our nervous systems.

Dissociation

If we have experienced acute Trauma, such as sexual abuse, then the body itself may not feel like a safe place to enter. We are embodied: we cannot escape. But this does not stop us trying.

One way we try to escape is by fragmenting from the body, known as dissociating. Dissociation is an energetic shift up into our head and out of connection with the body, so that we feel less. This is an instinctual ANS response that helps us survive traumatic or stressful situations. When we have experienced trauma, we may have a tendency to dissociate more readily, which perpetuates the constriction of our feelings. However, it is not only trauma survivors that dissociate. In our modern technological world, many of us have become 'walking heads' who do not fully feel our sensate aliveness.

Dissociation is a natural survival strategy, so it is not a 'bad' thing. But in the long term, being dissociated is detrimental to our health, because it means we are cut off from the fullness of our experience. Whilst this might keep us distanced from difficult feelings, it also makes us less available to the good feelings in life as well. It can also result in a poor sense of our own boundaries, because when we are disembodied, it is difficult to feel what is okay for us and what is not.

For many years, I have facilitated women to befriend and reconnect with their bodily sensations again. It takes time to learn to feel again, to begin to trust our own bodies and process the feelings and memories that arise as we do. But the more we can feel the body, the more consciously attuned we become to our own needs, patterns, creativity, desires and, importantly, what is not okay for us. Our wounds are part of Ereshkigal's moan that calls us back to ourselves.

Descending Back into the Body

Our personalities, how we communicate, what we show and what we hide about ourselves is, to a large extent, shaped by our relational experiences in childhood. The ways we learned to be loved and fit in with the world around us help define who we become. The heroine's journey is a process of becoming more aware of that shaping and how it affects the way we move through life. As we descend, we develop a growing awareness of our wounds and begin to notice the ways we have adapted and defended ourselves to compensate. For example, if we witnessed an act of violence in childhood and we wanted to scream, but it wasn't safe to, we probably held in the scream and held our breath. And twenty years later, on some level, we might still be holding our breath. Somatic Experiencing Practitioner, educator and author Kimberly Ann Johnson, compares the imprint of our old wounds to a scratch in a vinyl record. Each time you try to play your song, it either jumps over the scratch or gets stuck. This is what happens with our unprocessed trauma: the energy gets trapped and impedes our capacity to orientate ourselves and meet life in the here and now. The descent is the journey to consciously encounter the stuck cycles, the scratches, the trauma...

Inanna goes to the underworld to reveal her whole song.

As we descend, Inanna, our conscious awareness, moves down into the embodied subconscious to shed light on what has been in the dark. When we can witness and begin to feel the patterns, the places where the record is scratched, then we can start to remember our original song and free the life energy trapped there. It doesn't mean the scratch will go away completely. Our imprints may never fully disappear, but we can become more familiar with them and discover a way to move beyond their stronghold. Similar to when we manually work on scar tissue in the physical body, with massage and care, the tissue can become more pliant again. It is still scar tissue, but it becomes more integrated and less tender and rigid. When Inanna goes to meet Ereshkigal she tends to the scratches and scars.

As we move through life, our wounding inevitably gets sifted to the surface of our awareness and then, like Inanna, we can choose to turn towards it, or not. For many years I was carrying a freeze in my system that would show up in sexual intimacy with my husband. I couldn't trace its source, but it was trauma. I was highly functioning in my day-to-day life and you wouldn't think I was someone who was holding trauma. But there was a significant freeze in my system that would cause shut down in me that was uncomfortable and upsetting. I have worked for years to recalibrate this pattern and a lot of it has thawed, but certain things can set it off again. Getting to know its shape and the shadow of the pattern was an essential part of my own heroine's journey that has liberated me to grow beyond the freeze. From my own experience and the work I have done with women,

*I believe all women living in patriarchy have some
form of small t trauma in our bodies.*

Dr Stephen Porges' polyvagal theory has evidenced how, as human mammals, we co-regulate each other and how important social interaction and facial, vocal and physical cues are for our sense of safety. I believe that living in a misogynistic society where it is commonplace for women to be attacked, verbally or physically, must affect some kind of trauma response in women's bodies. Every time I go walking in the woods, every time I have to walk alone at night, every time I get cat-called, every time I go to a wedding and all the speeches are made by men, every time I get a letter addressed to Mrs J. Mountain, every time people refer to my children's toys as "he" as a given and every time another girl gets murdered on her way home from a friend's, I know that I live in an environment dominated by men, that holds an inherent disrespect for women.

Accommodation and the Female Nervous System

As Peter Levine, the founder and pioneer of Somatic Experiencing, states, *"If someone in your own group is threatening you, you may first try to 'make nice' before resorting to fighting or fleeing."* Accommodation is a natural human response to threat or conflict and it is an efficient one, as it can prevent a situation escalating. But I wonder exactly how much of women's creative energy is spent accommodating in the male-dominated environment, and what we could achieve if this was not such a preoccupation in our daily lives.

Unhealthy accommodation (sometimes referred to as *fawning*) of inappropriate male behaviour has been a huge part of my life. The degree to which I have accommodated others, particularly men, runs so deep it has taken literally decades of work to uncover it in my body. And since I continue to live in a patriarchy, I continue to have to do the work of flushing it out of my system repeatedly. For women without my privilege, things are significantly worse still. This accommodation of men to avoid unwanted attention or violence becomes a 'natural' part of our existence as women. But we seem to be realising more and more that it is not natural, normal or acceptable. It can be incredibly painful to wake up to how we have been victims of this.

Many studies of trauma assume that nervous system responses are gender neutral, but Kimberly Ann Johnson's work on the female nervous system challenges this. Unsurprisingly, the male norm has been assumed to be the female norm, giving us a misrepresentative picture of our own biology. In her book, *Call of the Wild*, Johnson notes that oestrogen is a bonding hormone which primes women to be more highly attuned to others. This is Mother Nature's clever way of helping women attune to our young. But, as she points out, the oestrogen in our bodies also means women are much more impacted by the social nervous system i.e. what happens in our environment, which, as she highlights, is both a superpower and can also mean that women have far more opportunity to be impacted by trauma. Until we grasp this, it can mean that we make decisions that previously we may not have been able to understand. She expounds,

> Women are confused as to why they went along with their doctor's recommendation when it didn't feel right, or stayed with an abusive partner. [...] Yes our conditioning to be 'good', 'nice' and not disruptive comes into play here, but so does our internal sense of survival, which tells us that we might not survive separation or conflict.

To know where a threat is by moving closer to it, is a survival strategy that many women have to employ. When we start to comprehend this, it can help dissolve shame and confusion about why we didn't respond to situations differently. It is so important that women's stories, experiences and unique biology are recognised, studied and discussed, so that we can more accurately understand our experiences and responses and bring Ereshkigal out of the dark. Otherwise, we simply try to adapt to male norms and then cannot understand why we keep feeling like we are failing.

Reconnecting to the Feminine

The uncovering of our own hidden stories can ignite an absolute craving for reconnection to the feminine, an insatiable hunger to intimately know our feminine ground of being. As I descended, I met with a ferocious longing inside myself, an obsessive desire for information and mirrors for my experience: I wanted to see myself and be witnessed in what was being revealed. I feasted on books, talks and poetry, really anything that helped anchor me in the wilderness of my experience, that gave me some reassurance in the unknown.

Reconnecting with our feminine ground of being is a very destabilising, disorientating experience. The heroine's journey inescapably lands us in the unknown. It is not linear, it is a necessary mess and there is no mediating authority along the way. We may look for one, but to do so is futile, because we are being returned to our senses, to the ancient knowing that is woven into all living things and ourselves. In order to arrive there, we must shed layers of conditioning, we must grieve, we must lose things along the way. The shiny veneer of the elevated masculine starts to chip away, and we land back in the wilderness of the feminine, that which has been denied and subjugated within us. In his book, *The Wild Edge of Sorrow,* a beautiful meditation on grief, Francis Weller states,

I see this work as soul activism, a form of deep resistance to the disconnected way in which our culture has conditioned us to live. Grief is subversive, undermining the quiet agreement to behave and be in control of our emotions. It is an act of protest that declares our refusal to live numb and small. There is something feral about grief, something outside of the ordained and sanctioned behaviours of our culture.

The descent also requires that we step outside of the ordained and sanctioned behaviours of our culture, and in doing so, we disrupt almost every known pattern of our personality. We embody these ordained and sanctioned behaviours in ways that we may know about and in lots of ways that we do not. Many of these patterns we take for granted as normal because they are all that we have known. The heroine's journey is a process of beginning to witness these patterns through fresh eyes, so that we can feel the way that they have subconsciously shaped our lives, choices and embodied experiences. Through this process we become a walking embodiment of change, the ripple effects of which move out from the inside of us into every interaction and relationship, eliciting change from the ground up and bringing the wisdom of our trauma into the light.

Chapter 4

REMEMBERING HER-STORY

"Women's stories have not been told. And without stories there is no articulation of experience. Without stories a woman is lost when she comes to make the most important decisions of her life. She does not learn to value her struggles, to celebrate her strengths, to comprehend her pain. Without stories she cannot understand herself. Without stories she is alienated from those deeper experiences of self and world that have been called spiritual or religious. She is closed in silence. The expression of women's spiritual quest is integrally related to the telling of women's stories. If women's stories are not told, the depths of women's souls will not be known.

Carol Christ, ***Deep Diving and Surfacing***

It's not news that we have been living his-story, but increasingly her-story is being revealed and prioritised, and it is changing the way we feel about the world. Women are hungry to hear about other women's lives. We want to see ourselves and our experiences reflected in the world. We want to hear women's hidden stories so that we can better locate ourselves in the landscape of womankind.

Though both male and non-binary characters feature in the Inanna-Ereshkigal myth, the leading characters are women. The myth is believed to have originated during a transitional period in time, when Sumeria was moving from a matrilineal structure to a patriarchy. I say matrilineal not matriarchal, because though in matrilineal societies wealth and name were passed through the female line of the family, there is little evidence to suggest that women dominated men in the culture. In her book, *The Chalice and the Blade*, Dr Riane Eisler suggests that matrilineal societies were much more egalitarian, with both men and women working in partnership rather than one sex dominating the other. In her work, Eisler highlights that the domination model we have been living under relies on a strong leader, a populist, one-man-solves-all hero. The kind that slays the dragon and vanquishes the wild feminine.

The Inanna-Ereshkigal myth is an antidote to this mythological rut. One of the most beautiful things I have come to know about the myth, is that it offers a complex framework for our inner and outer relationships that fosters compassion, empathy and a willingness to not know. Following the life/death/life cycle, it offers a potent embodied pathway into human complexity and connection that ultimately leads us back towards enduring love.

The inner core of patriarchal culture is estrangement, the estrangement of mind from body, men from women, thought from feeling, humans from earth.

Rosemary Reuther, *Goddess and the Divine Feminine*

The estrangement of patriarchal society manifests in a split from the wholeness of our experience. Domination is valued and encouraged over and above partnership and collaboration: men dominate women; humans dominate the Earth; white bodies dominate bodies of colour; heteronormativity dominates homosexuality and so on. And internally, we dominate parts of ourselves to fit into those societal ideals. As Eisler states,

The way that we structure the most fundamental of all human relations has a profound effect on every one of our institutions, on our values, and on the direction of our cultural evolution, particularly whether it will be peaceful or warlike.

Domination or Partnership?

Inanna and Ereshkigal have been at war inside of us. But we have the power to end this domination, to allow our own complexity and become more tactile to the nuances and subtleties of our beingness. When we do this internally, it affects how we relate to the world around us. The *way we structure the most fundamental of all human relations* also impacts the stories we tell and the stories we live. For many years, I thought the answer to our problems was the rise of the feminine. But I now realise that a dominator society could just as easily be matriarchal or patriarchal. Whereas, the Inanna-Ereshkigal myth teaches partnership, a paradigm that I feel holds valuable lessons for our time. As we start to deconstruct the inbuilt white privilege in our society and embrace all people, regardless of sexual orientation, religious beliefs, or other differences, I feel a partnership society would not only benefit women but would be more inclusive of all people, because in a partnership model, diversity is not equated with either inferiority or superiority. Partnership societies tend to be much less hierarchic and authoritarian.

The Hero's Journey

The hero's journey, as made popular by the work of Joseph Campbell, focuses on the ascent out into the world. Although in current times the term hero is used in a more gender-neutral way, many of our mythologies and stories based on the hero's map traditionally have had a male protagonist. Some writers, such as Sarah Nicholson and Mary Condren, have criticised Campbell's work for being too male-centric and omitting the intricacies and nuances of the female archetypal journey. As Condren discusses, "In their present form the myths are often blatant patriarchal propaganda extolling the virtues of a warrior society." Furthermore, in these mythologies women often lose their agency, as Nicholson explores,

As flesh, Woman loses her agency and it is the male who retains it, as well as the ability to act as hero. Woman disappears and is replaced by symbol because she is not fully allowed her subjectivity. Thus it becomes starkly clear why mythological figures of Woman are marked as non-heroic. Woman has been positioned as the purely phyllogenic source material (ripe, passive flesh) that has silently enabled the 'dazzling exploits' of the ontogenic male.

In the heroine's journey Inanna and Ereshkigal are active, subjective, female protagonists: Inanna chooses to descend rather than being taken. The agency of women in the story is a radical shift from the Persephones of our well-known mythologies, who are initiated by male protagonists. This agency feels important and enlivening to me.

The Heroine's Journey –
a feminine archetypal path

In 1990, driven by her desire to know specifically how women experience the hero's journey, Maureen Murdock wrote a paradigm-changing book about the heroine's journey. Within it, she explores what a mythological map of the archetypal feminine journey looks like and how it differs from the more widely-known hero's quest. She discusses in detail what it is like for a woman who spends a life living predominantly from her hero (masculine) energy.

The boon of success leaves these women overscheduled, exhausted, suffering from stress related ailments, and wondering how they got so off-track. This was not what they had bargained for when they first pursued achievement and recognition. The image they held of the view from the top did not include sacrifice of body and soul. In noticing the physical and emotional damage incurred by women on this heroic quest, I have concluded that the reason they are experiencing so much pain is that they chose to follow a model that denies who they are.

Murdock highlights how the models we live by in a patriarchal society prioritise masculine energy, which is much more linear than cyclical. Masculine dominance is so normalised that we often don't even recognise what is being denied within us. We have largely lost touch with the reverence for our natural rhythms and connectedness, to the detriment of all humankind and the Earth. Patriarchy has exiled the deep feminine at huge cost to us all. Feminist author and civil rights activist Audre Lorde said, "The Master's tools will never dismantle the Master's house". I believe that Ereshkigal's moan is a call to find a different way, one that reflects and honours the feminine, in all her shades and intricacy. So, it is towards our own moans, griefs, pains and bodies that we must go to uncover what we have forgotten.

Thirty years on from Murdock's writing, although there has been some significant change, women's bodily experiences and stories continue to get lost in translation within a male-dominated landscape. The consequence being that females are constantly accommodating paradigms that are not created for our benefit or anatomy. These narratives carry the nutrients of our cultural ideals.

But how nutritious are our dominant stories for women?

Popularised patriarchal heroes' journeys tend to see the hero killing or dominating the feminine: kidnapping and raping Persephone, beheading Medusa, exiling Circe... I question if this is the best way to be human? What is lost in this amputation of the feminine?

The Inanna-Ereshkigal myth does the opposite: Inanna goes to meet Ereshkigal, to be with her and enter a new partnership with the dark parts of the feminine. The heroine's journey is not a story of conquering or domination, it is about the complexity of relationship through which we can remember a different way of being. For too long, our lives have been directed towards the linear pursuit of success and achievement. Getting somewhere higher and better is what we are encouraged to do; but this paradigm is unsustainable.

His-story is not ending well.

The underworld journey is the antidote to the popularised hero's quest outwards: it calls us back down into our bodies, our relationships and our roots. It is significant to me that Covid, which I see as a collective initiation, did not happen 'out there' but in here, in our homes and bodies. Unless we were working on frontline services, we were held in our homes in an unprecedented way. As a result, many people descended into themselves in ways that busy life can stymie.

We are in uncharted territory and I feel that the map of the heroine's journey might help. Just as the layers of Inanna's upperworld identity are removed in her descent, so must we collectively slough off the layers that we have outgrown and seek other ways to be. This can seem like an impossibly huge task. So, we begin with the personal. If we listen to the knock at the door, the moan within, what is calling us? What is lying underneath the layers of our consciousness that society has encouraged us to bury?

A reflection on your relationship with the Feminine?

What does the word feminine mean to you?

How do you embrace the feminine? How do you reject the feminine?

What are your favourite heroines' stories?

Who are your favourite female role models/inspiration?

What inspires you about them? What specific qualities inspire you about them?

Which females do you dislike? What specific qualities do you dislike in them? What do you reject about them?

Anything else that has come up for you in this enquiry?

Sexual Assault and the #MeToo of the Descent

One aspect of women's experience that has been kept in shadow within our society is the abuse of women and girls. Violence towards women and girls has become a normal part of our culture. When women are murdered or raped, there is a whole conversation about what they were wearing, whether they did 'all the right things', as if, if they hadn't, it would somehow justify the perpetration. The #MeToo movement started by Tarana Burke, exposed millions of stories about the sexual abuse and harassment that people, and particularly women, experience. #MeToo stories spread across the internet like wildfire, oxygenating the magnitude of just how many women are subjected to inappropriate and invasive behaviour. This breaking of silence was a powerful moment in recent her-story that illustrates just how important empathy, solidarity and visibility are to help us recognise and break cycles of abuse. I spoke to artist and author Sivani Mata Francis about her descent,

"When I was eleven my grandmother died and that was my first big death. I was super close to her. But in some ways there was a sense of not fully going into the grief space because I felt my mum needed support. So I was not allowing myself to have the full descent and this has been a pattern for me. My godmother then died when I was fourteen, she was my closest adult in the world, and then my father died when I was seventeen. So, there was one loss after the other and a kind of like burying my feelings so as not to fully be in that grief space. Not surrendering, not shedding the layers that needed to be shed. It was a real holding back of that. Eventually, that manifested in some quite severe skin issues, because of me burying things. The grief was looking for another way out. In relation to the Inanna story, it was literally a layer of something on me that I needed to shed. With eczema and psoriasis, it's like the skin was actually doing what my emotional and mental capacity couldn't get to – my skin was a physical embodiment of it.

That process of denial, of loss, led me to do silly things as a teenager. I had lots of one-night stands, because I wanted to have the closeness but I didn't want to experience the loss. In a one-night stand, it's like, you don't dive deep enough to get that experience of loss. But that culminated in me being raped and then there were years of dealing with what I'd done. Definitely a sense of self blame, for both experiences – of me looking for it and it coming knocking on my door."

Feelings of self-blame are often carried by women who experience sexual assault. Sadly, this is exacerbated by cultural narratives that still tend to put the onus on women's behaviour, rather than focusing on the perpetrator. #MeToo has encouraged women to speak up about their hidden stories and to look at sexual perpetrations from the viewpoint of women and girls. When we realise that our personal stories are actually a collective experience and a systemic problem, it can strengthen our convictions and encourage us to admit what happened to us, thereby relieving ourselves of the shame and blame. As Clarissa Pinkola Estés names,

The way to change a tragic drama back into a heroic one is to open the secret, speak of it to someone, write another ending, examine one's part in it and one's attributes in enduring it. These learnings are in equal parts pain and wisdom. The having lived through it is a triumph of the deep and wild spirit.

I feel women have, on some level, been stuck in a *tragic drama* for the duration of patriarchal life. Keeping the experiences and feelings that come with sexual violation underground impacts us in all sorts of ways. Now is the time for change. Language has power. The stories we live and tell literally shape our world and sense of self. The telling of our stories can help us to transform our tragedies into gold. I have also experienced this through poetry. When I hear a story or poem that speaks to my experience, I feel met and immediately less alone. The stories we tell can provide a much-needed response to Ereshkigal's moan. This response helps us symbolise our inner experience in the outer world and can be a way to bring Ereshkigal out of the dark.

But, unfortunately, when we speak of the *secret* of our abuses, it is still all too common for us not to be heard or taken seriously. Misogynistic culture makes it very difficult for women to speak up about abuse. Like the Sky Gods and Dumuzi, there is a part of every single one of us that does not want *to examine our part in the tragedy* or look at the pain of it. One of the reasons that I feel it is so imperative to hear this myth, at this time, is because it can be a companion and guide, as we walk off the beaten track and face what comes as a result. It is a story that recognises the courage it takes to enter the underworld and encourages us to keep going.

Telling our stories is a way to build communities that provide new homes of belonging and support, as we navigate the choppy waters of change. As Carol Christ says, *"the expressions of women's spiritual quest are integrally related to the telling of women's stories."* Encountering the Inanna-Ereshkigal myth consecrated my own life story. This helped me transform difficulty into gold, not only for myself, but in the creation of work that now helps other people as they navigate their heroine's journeys. But initially, we may find ourselves *knocking on the door of the wrong gods*. Sivani Mata's story speaks to this,

> "Many years after I was raped, I had been in this space of courage and reflection supported by my yoga practice and so I told my yoga teacher what had happened to me. It was kind of like the first time I had been able to voice, 'this is what happened'. He did not respond in the best of ways, and I had a forced sexual experience with him which I didn't want or expect – that sort of re-traumatised me again."

#MeToo stories do not just happen in 'bad' situations, they regularly happen in the situations that we least expect, and most sexual violations are perpetrated by people we know and trust. Sadly, yoga and spiritual communities are also places where abuse happens. From the Catholic Church, to therapy rooms, to yoga studios, to the film industry, to the police force, #MeToo stories continue to trickle out of all areas of society. Misogyny appears in all places. This was an important turning point for Sivani Mata as she continues,

"That journey led me to Uma Dinsmore-Tuli, where I found a safe space in feminine holding and a process of doing women's work and then assisting on the courses and coming more into that space of learning to listen. I had been doing three hours of yoga practice, same thing, every day, quite a rigid Hatha practice, which was beautiful in some ways, and I loved it, but I also got burnt out. I got seriously bad anaemia.

The coming out of that, was coming to Uma and learning that I can do different things on different days, different parts of my cycle need different attention. I had read *Red Moon* by Miranda Gray before coming to Uma, so was starting to get into this consciousness of paying attention to my cycles. But the work with Uma, this rhythm of different responses at different times was super important to me.

And then, through that work, hearing other women's stories and the #MeToo of that was really important. Hearing stories, not only with sexual trauma, but with grief, with every aspect of life and knowing that we are not alone. And that's important because with grief or a trauma, sometimes there is a fear…fear to speak out, because you feel like you're the only one and you don't want to be singled out as a mess, or the one who 'should have known better,' or the only one that 'got into that kind of trouble'. There is something very liberating in knowing that we're all in it together and that's life."

As Sivani Mata highlights, sharing stories can be such a powerful experience. If we do not find a home for our stories, then they might remain buried inside of us and never see the light of day, meaning we may be tempted to pass off our experiences as nothing more than failures or mistakes. This can breed a stifling sense of shame as Sivani Mata articulates, a fear that it's 'our fault' and that we are the 'only ones'. Shame perpetuates the split between Inanna, who becomes our elevated or idealised self,[*] and Ereshkigal who continues to be hidden and denied. As Sivani Mata concludes,

> "To bring it back to the beginning of my story, of not allowing myself to go into that grief because of the fear of where that would leave me. I now know that it's vital, to dive into it and surrender. We have to end up like Inanna, being strung up and naked. We have to strip everything, because only then can we really rise from it. Without the stripping down to the truth of it, of the reality of our existence, who we are in that moment, whatever we have buried is just hovering and continuously coming back to say, 'Hey, remember me?'…If we bury it we don't learn anything."

Being seen compassionately, in our experience, can diffuse the cloak of shame and allow us to bring light to our experience, to grow through it and create a bridge between the parts of ourselves that have been estranged. As Sivani Mata wisely points out, then our wounds become our teachers. In women's circles, our shared experiences actually become the glue that creates bonds of connection unlike anything else. When we dare to reveal Ereshkigal, we can begin to feel and admit both her pain *and* her power and wisdom. Rather than splitting off from or trying to suppress our feelings we can move towards wholeness. This process frees what has been exiled, back into the fullness of life, so that eventually we can rise rooted in all that we are.

---

[*] That being all the ways that we consciously and subconsciously pretend to be something that we are not, in an attempt to avoid unhappiness or rejection. I first came across this idea through the teachings of the Pathwork via Kim Rosen. See References for more.

Chapter 5

INTRODUCING INANNA, THE GREAT GODDESS

In ancient Sumer, Inanna as a goddess of sexuality, fertility and power was worshipped by men and women alike. Artefacts found from this time seem to point to worship of the Goddess and menstrual blood as a part of praise for the life-giving rivers of the womb. As patriarchal culture began to take over, this was lost. In *Dancing in the Flames – the Dark Goddess in the Transformation of Consciousness*, Marion Woodman and Elinor Dickson discuss,

> *Whereas they had once taken power from nature through bone, feathers and blood, now they sought to exert power over nature. All the powers that had been an expression of the Great Mother were now transferred to the Sun. Humanity moved from polytheism to monotheism. Nature in this patriarchal paradigm, was seen as something to be controlled and dominated.*

This narrative, of praising the sun, praising the masculine energetic qualities of doing, producing and knowing, have become more and more deeply embedded in our Western cultural paradigms. We can see this reflected across our systems and institutions. History is a story told by men, with men at the centre.

What If?

What if it had been the Mother, the
Daughter and the Holy Spirit?
How different might things be then,

if women only had their natural limits?
Blood revered as a superpower,
as beautiful and welcomed and earthly as a flower.
Childbirth, if chosen, a sacred rite of passage.
Midwives as holy women,
Crones as the wisdom cup.
A sisterhood, a sisterhood.
Nature as Queen and ageing as a privilege.
What if it had been the Mother, the
Daughter and the Holy Spirit?
How different might things be then?

The spirit of Sumerian culture, as a pre-patriarchal society, was fundamentally different to anything we have ever known. Therefore, a myth that arose from this cultural landscape holds in its very foundations a different embodied teaching of what is possible for us, here and now. Other parts of the poem, as translated by Wolkstein and Kramer, depict in great detail and have a sense of celebration of Inanna's sexual desire and expression. She is an empowered, sexually liberated, loved goddess, whole in her own right, without having to be attached to a masculine god-figure – we explore this more in Gates Six and Seven. In one passage Inanna is described as,

"*...a maid*
As tall as heaven,
as wide as earth,
As strong as the foundations of the city wall"

Even before Inanna descends, she is strong, empowered and she is the protagonist of her own story: a mature, sexual, sovereign being, who knows that in order to embody her wholeness, she must be initiated. When she is asked to submit, it is to the laws of the underworld, Ereshkigal's realm.

This is the feminine submitting to the feminine.

I believe we can all embody this Queendom. But sexual and spiritual maturity that is rooted in the deep feminine, is not the norm in our culture. Far from recognising our heroines' journeys as a divine rite of passage, in the spirit of our times, many women entering this initiation actually believe there is something wrong with them. I hear women say things like: "*I wish I could get my rage under control*", "*I wish I could just get over this*", "*My partner thinks I have gone mad*", "*I really need to get a grip*" or "*I wish I could just stop feeling so emotional*". When we stop being able to comply, the default position is often to assume that *we* are at fault. On the contrary, I would strongly suggest that these symptoms are not wrong. They are a call from Ereshkigal, and she is trying to show us how to hear her. But it can be deeply uncomfortable to do so.

The descent happens when something unequivocally gives
in inside us and we finally say yes, I will listen.

The descent is an embodied reversal of the patriarchal norms and values that we have been taught to inhabit. It is a reawakening of the ancient feminine within. It feels dangerous because for hundreds of years it was.

The red thread of our matriarchal lines and stories have largely been dominated and buried by patriarchy. There was a period spanning approximately five hundred years between the twelfth and seventeenth centuries where women remotely connected to their feminine power and anyone who supported them, were brutally tortured and burned at the stake for witchcraft. It is thought that many female healers, midwives and wise women were murdered in this violent period of history.

The 'Witches' were the ones who had developed extensive knowledge of herbs and anatomy... The disappearance of the Midwives in the 17-18th century, created an in road for the non-professional male practitioners – the 'Barber Surgeons'. They led the way in England claiming technical superiority over midwives on the basis of their use of obstetric forceps, which were legally classified as a surgical instrument and women were legally barred from surgical practice. This changed the neighbourly midwifery service into a lucrative business and was taken over by the Physicians in the 18th century. A similar story happened worldwide and mostly remains the same.

Jane Hardwicke Collings, *Herstory*

This was a powerful moment of physical severance in our her-story. I believe we are still healing from the trauma of those losses and persecutions to this day. Many of the attitudes woven into Christianity and medicine are rooted in this period of history. Even now, in many parts of the world, women's wisdom, ways and stories still have to go underground for fear of the violence of male oppression.

One of the many costs of this is that without our female lineages and stories, when we want to step off the well-furrowed track of men, we can feel utterly lost. For me, it was like stepping into an abyss of the unknown. Like so many women surviving in patriarchy, nearly all the women around me were living predominantly from an adaptation to the masculine. What I was desperate to discover was how to follow the feminine energy in me and how to hold other women as they healed their connection to their wounded feminine. As historian Gerda Lerner articulates,

Men develop ideas and systems of explanation by absorbing past knowledge and critiquing and superseding it. Women, ignorant of their own history do not know what women before them had thought and taught. So, generation after generation, they struggle for insights others already had before them, resulting in the constant inventing of the wheel.

The heroine's journey is the path to remembering the red thread of our matrilineal line and our cyclical wisdom, so that we can begin to reclaim our exiled feminine energy and let it guide and nourish us. I don't think it's a mistake that women's circles are of increasing popularity at this time: we are hungry for circles of connection and we are creating them. For almost a decade now, I have held women's sacred spaces and have seen first-hand the positive impact that shared stories and community can have. The scarcity of women's stories means that women have had to deal with so much that has not been spoken about, alone. This has kept us separated, in the dark and insecure. But increasingly, we are bringing more and more of *her* stories into the light to be seen, felt and heard. We need the whole spectrum of women's stories to be revealed, so that we can inspire and inform each other, grieve together, and help guide each other forwards.

Where Do Our Heroines' Stories Live and What Can They Teach Us?

There are an increasing number of women-led books, films and creative projects emerging in this time of reclaiming and remembering women's stories. One of the forerunners of this movement, Clarissa Pinkola Estés' book, *Women Who Run with the Wolves*, offers a bible of female mythology. Lucy H. Pearce (whose experiences are shared in this book) writes books that focus on women's stories and experiences. Her publishing house, Womancraft Publishing, which published this book, was set up in 2014 specifically to publish books written by women, for women. Trista Hendren, who you have met already, founded Girl God Books at about the same time. The Awakening Women Institute offers sadhanas on feminine mythology and spirituality. There are also now many popular retellings of myths from female perspectives, such as Madeline Miller's captivating novel, *Circe*. Even Disney-Pixar have an increasing catalogue of heroines' stories like *Brave* and *Moana*. And the hugely successful Crowdfunded, *Goodnight Stories for Rebel Girls*, is an encyclopaedia of stories about inspiring, real life heroines. This book was the catalyst for many other books and podcasts that followed about notable women, whose achievements and discoveries were previously buried in history, unnamed and uncelebrated. We are slowly resurrecting our heroines.

If the stories of women's lives are not told, if women and girls are never the protagonists of our stories, then we lose a sense of our own location and perpetuate the notion that girls and women are not worthwhile or important. In 2016, *Time* magazine compiled a list of the "Best 100 children's books of all time": only fifty-three of those books had females that speak. Thankfully, this is changing. In 2004, actress Geena Davis founded the Geena Davis Institute on Gender in Media. Her mission was to provide research that shows the gender imbalance in our media and influence change,

The stories that we choose to tell in entertainment media send a specific message about who matters most in our culture. In order to bring about a global culture change, it is especially important that children see diverse, intersectional representations of characters in media to reflect the population of the world—which is half female and very diverse— and avoid unwittingly instilling unconscious bias in them.

For so long, women have been the objects, not the subjects, of our stories. In addition, when women do feature, we have often occupied a supporting role to the leading male, rather than the lead itself. Or we have been allowed to be some things and not others: a woman seeking romance with a desirable male, an evil witch, or a victim. Stories help to define what girls can aspire to be and how girls are expected to behave. Relating this to the Inanna-Ereshkigal myth, Inanna symbolises the parts of us that are welcomed by society, Ereshkigal the parts that are not. Ereshkigal holds the parts that the upperworld loves to hate. She serves as a warning to women who are too wild, too sexual, too rageful, too outspoken, that they will be exiled if they do not keep those parts of themselves down. Similar splitting of female archetypes can be seen in common cultural tropes such as the virgin and whore, the beautiful young woman and the old hag, the evil mother and the victimised daughter. In our Western Christian religion, the Virgin Mary was the uplifted chaste mother, whilst Mary Magdalene was cast as the whore.

When we look at depictions of the Goddess in other parts of the world, the feminine is not so one-dimensional. She can be simultaneously fierce, fecund and benevolent. For example, the Hindu goddess, Durga, rides a tiger and wields weapons, she is fierce and boundaried. The Sheela na Gig, interpreted by some researchers to be an ancient Irish goddess of birth and death, is an archetype akin to Ereshkigal. The Sheela na Gig holds open her vulva with her own hands and used to be commonly found in the stonework of Irish churches and in some other places across Europe. Through her open vulva she invites us to be receptive to what is birthing from within us, and what is dying.

There are, in fact, hundreds of goddesses from all different cultures and traditions. But our Western society still sits under the dominance of our monotheistic church-based religion, which traditionally holds God, the disembodied Father, at the centre. Meanwhile, the Goddess and the feminine have been relegated to the edges of our awareness. Only the 'desirable' parts are invited into societal space and the other more complex parts, like Ereshkigal, are still exiled, denigrated or have been buried altogether.

It is our job to rebirth and reclaim her as a part of us.

As feminist, theologian and author Carol Christ describes,

The symbol of the Goddess has much to offer women who are struggling to be rid of the 'powerful, pervasive, and long-lasting moods and motivations' of devaluation of female power, denigration of the female body, distrust of female will, and denial of the women's bonds and heritage that have been engendered by patriarchal religion. As women struggle to create a new culture in which women's power, bodies and bonds are celebrated, it is natural that the Goddess would re-emerge as a symbol of the newfound beauty, strength and power of women.

The multiplicity of the Goddess can be an invitation to be all that we are. She does not have to be this or that, she can be many things: she is matter, she is divine, she holds many energies, she is complex, sometimes contradictory, and importantly, she can be wild.

Journalling enquiry on your relationship with the Goddess(es)

What is your relationship with the Goddess? Let your pen flow, even if it does not seem to make sense, and see what comes up. Here are some questions to help you.

If you have a favourite goddess who is she?

What is it that draws you to her?

Who knows about your relationship with the Goddess? Is it central to your life or more personal?

How do you include or exclude this part of you?

Conversely, if you do not have a relationship with goddesses I invite you to write about that. What do you associate with goddesses?

What does not resonate with you?

How do you feel about this enquiry?

Chapter 6

CALLING IN THE WITNESS – MEETING NINSHUBUR

In life, our primary witness is often (not always) our mother. As our first loyal witness, when we *goo goo,* hopefully she *goo goos* and when we *gaa gaa,* she *gaa gaas.* Just as when the *kugarra* and the *galatur* empathise with Ereshkigal, seemingly simple empathic social responses are profoundly important for us as infants and adults. In the Inanna-Ereshkigal myth, the necessity of the witness is personified a number of times, which is testament to the importance of being witnessed in our lives, particularly in difficult times. As infants, we rely on these primary loving interactions from our caregivers to thrive. Through this relationship we begin to develop our communication and our social brain, which forms the foundation for how we communicate in our lives. We learn to notice social cues, facial expressions and read the movements of others and through these interactions, this witnessing and being witnessed, we develop the pre-frontal cortex of the brain. Over time, we also learn to witness our inner state in relationship to our outer environment and measure our responses accordingly. The pre-frontal cortex is an essential mediator in that process and could be thought of as the seat of our inner Ninshubur, our inner witness. As Inanna's handmaiden, Ninshubur symbolises the part of us that stays above ground, whilst another part of us, Inanna, descends. Ninshubur, is the one inside us who may still be able to seek help and articulate some of what is happening to us, whilst another part of us is underground, immersed in the subconscious process. As author and Jungian analyst Sylvia Brinton Perera names,

Ninshubur for me, is the model of woman's deepest, reflective-of-the-Self, priestess function, one which operates as simple executive of the Self's commands, often when the soul is most threatened.

I think it's quite beautiful to think of her as the "priestess" of the temple of us. The one who holds the integrity of our inner structure, whilst the other parts of us are being de-constructed. In this respect, the witness inside us is essential for our integration, survival and ultimately, our sanity. Even though most of our energy is below ground, she is the part of us who gets the necessary stuff of life done in the upperworld whilst we are in the underworld. Some of us may not work, or are so incapacitated for a time that we are signed off work, but for many people this is not possible.

A common theme for the women I interviewed, is that normal life was continuing whilst they were in the underworld. I believe that Ninshubur is the one that makes that possible. Despite the fact that we are sitting in the wreckage of our crumbling identity, she stays loyal to our quest. Whilst some of those nearest to us may not be able to bear the changes taking place within us, she has an unswerving commitment to the part of us that has gone below – her role is paramount. As author and founding director of the Institute for Integrative Bodywork and Movement Therapy, Linda Hartley names,

When we journey within there are many depths to be encountered, but Ereshkigal's realm is the deepest we may descend to with the possibility of safe return; beyond that it is full-blown psychosis or actual physical death. The fine line that discriminates initiation from psychosis on this journey is essentially one of consciousness and the meaning we are able to give to the experience; this is dependent on the many levels of holding...the descent to the underworld is a sacred journey, endured for sacred purpose. We may not know the purpose, but we feel it in our blood and in our bones.

The way that we were parented has a big effect on the development of our internal witness, our inner Ninshubur. Their external voice, on some level becomes our internal voice, for better or worse. Not all the scripts we internalise in childhood are positive. We can begin to unpack the scripts we have internalised in therapy or spiritual work. For example, the idea that we must *always* put others' needs before our own is a script that, if followed to an extreme, leads us to have poor boundaries and become a doormat. But if we can begin to work with that script and be supported to witness and feel how damaging it is, we can begin to make different choices. An inherent part of the descent is to learn to notice the scripts that we have internalised and how these might be useful or detrimental to our behaviour, choices and how we witness ourselves.

The social context in which we live also has a huge influence on these scripts. As women living in misogynistic culture, there are many scripts that we adopt that do not serve us. A key aspect of our descent is waking up to these, bringing them to consciousness, and slowly changing our relationship to our internal voices. Eventually, Ninshubur can become a supportive and compassionate inner witness, more than a critical voice. As Sivani Mata named, when she yielded to the descent and began to learn how to witness herself there, the grief that she had been so afraid to surrender to became her teacher and eventually her strength.

Earlier I mentioned implicit memories, memories held in the body. Our inner witness can remember how to track the body to find our way into the feelings and energy of the somatic imprints that we hold. Therapy, yoga and other movement practices can provide a place where we listen, feel and allow what arises in the body to show us what is in the dark of our awareness and how to be with it. This is a form of self-witnessing.

In day-to-day life, there are some cues that can help. One way that we avoid Ereshkigal is by rejecting or overriding her 'natural' or 'animal response'. So, for example, we are tired, but we have a deadline and so we overwork and push through. Then when we get home and our partner offers to make us a tea, we bite their head off because we are so frazzled. Or conversely, if our bodies are craving rest and our inner critic rears up, telling us that we are 'being lazy' (this is another example of a script). The arrival of the inner critic is always a key sign that we are defending a vulnerability or avoiding a need. Both of these are examples of the internal splitting between Inanna and Ereshkigal: what is happening in the body, versus what we think 'should' be happening, do not match. When Ninshubur wakes up to this, we can begin to actually listen for what is happening underneath our initial responses and discover the shadow – the energy of Ereshkigal – hidden there.

Another example occurs in the myth, when Ereshkigal meets Inanna and all of her rage comes roaring up. Under the rage is the unmet pain that Ereshkigal has not been able to admit. Rage is Ereshkigal's first defence. Uncontrollable outbursts of rage often come with unprocessed trauma and PTSD. Under that anger is the wound that is craving empathy.

So how do we work with these patterns and start to track the deeper layers of our experience?

The first thing is to notice. A check list of red flags might include:

- I am irritable, tetchy or defensive

- I become aware that I am overreacting to a situation

- I feel rage or anger and am not sure why

- I feel overwhelmed

- I feel like I need to escape even though I know rationally that I am not under immediate threat from anything

- I am overthinking and cannot switch off my thoughts

- I am saying yes when I mean no, or no when I mean yes

- I have lost my voice and cannot find the words I need to speak.

There are more variations that can crop up, but these ones are common to many people. When we notice these responses arise there is a simple exercise that can help us to bring Ninshubur, our inner witness, in to help us.

Witnessing ourselves

1. Slow down enough to pause and observe your responses.

2. Take a moment to ask yourself, what is the need that is arising?

3. Notice your body. What sensations can you feel? Is there a voice inside that is not being honoured? Can you take a deep breath? If you can't feel your body, that is something to notice. You could massage or tap your arms, hands and feet to help bring sensation back.

4. If you can locate a need, check in if there is any judgement about this need? If there is, breathe into it, feel it, maybe journal around it. The inner critic's presence is a classic defence mechanism. Bring the critic home by asking what she needs.

---

5. Ask yourself, how can you tend to the need inside? Do you need to ask someone else for some help?

6. If you have been able to identify what is playing out, see if you can make one small step towards what you need. Remember you don't have to be perfect. Small, digestible steps and a lot of compassion is what is needed.

7. Complete the listening exercise by giving thanks to yourself and your inner Ninshubur for taking this time to witness what is here.

Note: if you cannot locate a need sometimes it can be because you require more time or support to access these vulnerable layers. Go slowly. Do the first three steps of the process as many times as necessary and see what emerges. Old patterns do not and should not change overnight. The most lasting change is often that which happens slowly. If you feel the urgency for immediate change, that too is something to notice and sit with.

Initially, this kind of practice is best explored with an external witness who can help us to hold what is coming up, such as a therapist or space-holder. A therapist can offer an empathic response that we may not yet be able to offer to ourselves, as the *kugarra* and *galatur* do for Ereshkigal in the story. Importantly, when we notice what the body says, we can begin to feel our own needs. As someone who has a tendency to focus on the needs of others, at times I still lose a sense of my own needs. To recognise this in itself can feel acutely vulnerable; to know we need something, but not know what, can be a big edge to meet. When we can bear to open to that vulnerability, we make a step towards Ereshkigal, a step towards finding out what is in shadow that we have not yet admitted. If what we are meeting inside has been buried for a long time, it is a good idea to seek out support as we go into the dark of our underworld.

To slow down and call in Ninshubur is a key step for all of us, so that we can be increasingly aligned with our own needs and integrity. Incongruence happens when what we are living does not align with the truth of what is inside of us. Incongruence relies on self-abandonment to be sustained, this is a key teaching of the descent and especially Gate Four. With the support of Ninshubur, we gradually begin to feel the pain of abandoning ourselves which enables us to change the pattern. Ninshubur plays a vital role in healing the rift between Inanna and Ereshkigal, because she interrupts the pattern of abandoning Ereshkigal again. She holds us as we turn towards our wounded self.

On an external level, Ninshubur can represent someone who we trust, who has the capacity to witness our descent. This role is often taken on by a therapist, teacher, elder, guide, friend or loved one. My Ninshuburs, women's initiatory guide, Jules Heavens and my spiritual teacher Kim Rosen, were essential for helping me to decipher what was happening and how to navigate it. They also modelled for me different ways of beholding and witnessing myself. Books and poetry were also a form of Ninshubur for me. I remember devouring poems as essential soul food, and finding this myth was a life-saving moment for me. Consecration is so essential for keeping us alive in the underworld. Books and myths are not dead objects, they are living Ninshuburs and can be vital lifelines as we descend.

Women's Circles as Ninshubur

The split between Inanna and Ereshkigal is also mirrored in our wounded sisterhood. When there are only a few seats at the patriarchal table, one way of surviving is to compete with each other, or dissociate from being female altogether. In patriarchy, women are often pitted against each other. But women who are awakening want company and to have the companionship of other women, as we revive the wild woman inside us that has been alone in exile for so long. In sacred circles, we can find the compassion, trust, love and solidarity that we may never have had with other women. This solidarity is much needed for our journey. The circle becomes a group of Ninshuburs who will bang the drum for us. Research has shown that women release oxytocin (known as the love hormone) when they sit together in circles. There can be a safety and an energy in all-female spaces that allows our bodies to open.

Women's circles can offer empathic witnessing and beholding that reinstates a sisterhood of support.

Many women who come to the circles that I hold arrive having not had good experiences of sisterhood. At school and in the workplace it is not unusual for women to be really nasty to each other and our media actively encourages this. But women's bodies are made to synchronise, and women living together often find that they bleed together on the dark moon and ovulate on the full moon (though not always in this rhythm). I had a vision when writing this book of a powerful blood tide created by the sea of the feminine, our wombs connecting us across the planet. But, like our actual seas, our wombs and blood tides have been polluted and mistreated and many of our wombs have never known sisterhood.

But we can remember.

A women's circle can be a place where we create a new paradigm of community and partnership. One that does not shame emotionality and difficulty, but supports us as we grieve our losses and celebrates us when we shine. Through sharing in circle, we begin to see how the wounds we carry are both deeply personal and archetypal – there is a medicine in that.

The Vital Need for Being Seen and Witnessed

The stuff of our heroines' journeys often happens behind closed doors, unwitnessed, in the fabric of our lives. The power of being witnessed in these experiences is essential. When we begin to compost the old identities and scripts that have helped us belong to the society/family/relationships/culture in which we have lived, it can feel totally obliterating. Without a witness, the landscape can feel unbearably desolate. One of the reasons I am writing this book is in the hope that it will be a Ninshubur for anyone who needs one, the way that Linda Hartley's book, *Servants of the Sacred Dream*, was for me.

I am so heartened to see that heroines' journeys are being dramatised more and more. In pioneering work such as Michaela Coel's *I May Destroy You* and even in mainstream children's films, such as *Frozen*, which follows Elsa's descent into the underworld of her own power that she has been told by her parents to suppress. As Elsa approaches maturity and her impending role as queen, these powers can no longer stay hidden and she has to find a way to integrate them.

She goes on a heroine's journey to meet her power, dissolve her fear and use the love she feels to integrate it. Her sister Anna is her witness, her Ninshubur, and sisterhood is the key to unlocking the love that dissolves the freeze around Elsa's power. In previous times, that role would have been filled by the prince.

In *I May Destroy You*, Michaela Coel takes an unflinching look at sexual abuse and the many ways that it infiltrates our culture and relationships. Inside this narrative we see the importance of the witness in her best friend, Terry, who stays beside her in the aftermath of sexual assault as she walks the messy path of bringing Ereshkigal out of the dark. Terry is her Ninshubur. In the final episode, Coel's character, a writer who has been struggling creatively since her assault, starts mapping the timeline of her story onto her bedroom wall with Post-it notes. As I watched this, I imagined her consciously seeing her own heroine's journey. I don't know if that is what Coel was intending (I would love to know!) but as she discovers the external map for her internal experience, her creativity starts to flow again and she rises back into her life. What makes this work even more powerful for me, is that Michaela Coel created and acted in it, after she was sexually assaulted herself. She used her creativity as a Ninshubur and a way to rise. We speak more about creativity as a witness in Gate Five. I see *I May Destroy You* as a powerful modern-day portrayal of the heroine's journey.

Journalling prompt: Ninshubur

Who (or what) are your key witnesses or supports in life? If you notice that you do not have any external witnesses, you might want to feel into what kind of Ninshubur you are longing for.

What qualities would she have? And where might you seek her out?

Chapter 7

THE SEVEN GATES OF THE DESCENT

In the myth of Inanna, the heroine descends through seven gates to the underworld. In her book, *Descent to the Goddess,* Sylvia Brinton Perera suggests that these seven gates can be related to the seven chakra points in the body from the crown of the head down to the pelvis. The chakras are most commonly approached in the hero's direction of lower to higher, mirroring the dominant ideological spiritual and secular pursuit of 'higher' knowledge and transcendence. In this case, chakra one is the root chakra, and we proceed upwards to chakra seven at the crown chakra and beyond. In the heroine's descent, we reverse the direction, moving from the crown as chakra one and descending down to the root as chakra seven and beyond. My whole being delights in this reversal. In our modern mind-led technological age, I feel we desperately need mythological and spiritual teachings that show us the way back down to Earth.

In order to honour the nature of the descent, I created a spiral map, to show the embodiment of the heroine's journey. I have chosen a spiral because when we are first born, as babies, we spiral out through the birth canal (unless caesarean born) and the heroine's journey is a rebirth. Additionally, I feel that a more linear pathway does not reflect the embodied experience of descent. Ultimately, to follow a linear path is to have some kind of rational control and coherence in an experience. Whereas, the heroine's path is disorientating and be-wild-ering, something more akin to walking through a dark bramble forest than on a concrete pavement. When we enter the integrity of our somatic experience, we have to feel our way forwards, we cannot purely think our way there. Though the descent is not linear, the provision of seven gates does provide an esoteric structure through which we can glean valuable insight. But in real life, we are unlikely to progress through the gates in such a consciously sequential manner. Much of the process happens subconsciously and moments of insight become like breadcrumbs on the path that provide essential morsels of nourishment along the way.

Entering the Landscape of Emotion

When we land in the body, we also land in our feelings: a fundamental part of the heroine's journey involves entering the emotional body. Having followed a patriarchal yoga lineage for over a decade, my emotional body had been negated within my practice, in favour of the calm rationality that often goes with the yoga persona. The emotional body, often called-out for being irrational, even hysterical, actually has a deep wisdom and emotional processing is a vital part of healing the injured cycles that have manifested through our traumas and wounding. The word *hysterical* originates from the Greek word for uterus and has derogatory associations rooted in female emotionality and anatomy. To be welcome at the table of patriarchy, women are often told not to become 'too emotional' and sadly many boys still don't cry. All the emotions we have curtailed, denied or suppressed must be met on the way down into the body. For me, when my emotional floodgates opened, it was such a relief. I could finally be a mess, not have to hold to form, or will, or even be rational. The underworld was a place where the small loomed large and feelings roamed like dragons: a place I could splurge and sound and melt.

This is the compost heap of our humanness, it is the
land of earthworms, musk and decay.

The experience I describe is totally at odds with teachings I had come across about the body, chakras and spirituality. The writings I encountered on these subjects were mostly conveyed through a clean academic tone and structure, that omitted any emotional colour: something that would speak to the Sky

Gods more than the Goddess. So many embodied practices prioritise equanimity within us, sometimes at the expense of authentic feeling. This can lead to a quietness, a politeness that does not allow the emotional body to be included or expressed. Obviously, when deep meditative states of peace organically appear in us, they are beautiful. But to raise this particular way up to be *the* way of being in the body, can be very confining. Even in the spiritual landscape there can be a dominator dynamic, where hierarchies of practice end up being another way that we strive to become more superior to others. In dualistic spiritual systems, one way of being is elevated as preferable to another. In this paradigm, at best we might learn good discipline, but at worst it may keep us from being with the truth and fullness of our experience.

The culmination of all the above meant that, for many years, embodied practice was not something that included emotion for me. I found the chakras to be an inaccessible construct that did not resonate with the feelings and experiences of my own body. So, I wondered if perhaps I wasn't quite feeling it right, or didn't fully understand it. But I *was* feeling and experiencing a lot. So I used to scour books, desperately looking for a description that resonated with something, anything, of how I was experiencing embodied awakening. But I found very little. This is how hierarchies of knowledge can disenfranchise us from our own body's wisdom.

Over two decades of yoga and embodied spiritual practice, I have come to discover that we all experience the chakras in everyday life whether we recognise it or not. They may at first seem esoterically removed from our day-to-day existence, but actually these energetic centres inform what we crave, what we prioritise and how the energy of our lives moves. The sensitivity to feel this consciously is something many of us lose touch with, but it is totally possible to reconnect to the subtle body and our cyclical wisdom, and *anyone* with the desire to do so can access it. I have beheld many women in the journey to reclaim their spirituality in a form that is rooted in the Earth, the body and our sensual and sexual selves. In the spaces that I hold emotional expression, when it arises, is included as a sacred vehicle to awakening. Often, we try to make the body tidy, we ask it to be obedient, clean and socially acceptable. But intimacy is necessarily messy and the heroine's journey holds intimacy at its core. Intimacy with what?

On the heroine's journey, we almost always begin in the
personal and end in the arms of the mystery.

Sacred Practices – building an altar

We are about to enter the descent and a sacred ritual that I find nourishing is building an altar. An altar is a symbol of what is sacred. It can also be an outer symbol of our inner life, an external anchor for our internal work. For me it is also a reassuring reminder that we are held by the mystery or the Goddess, something beyond what we can fully know or name. It is also a practice of devotion. An altar can be a place that we visit or pray to, something tangible that can help us bring focus to that which is intangible but always present, in nature and in life. I find rituals like this very supportive in the face of all that I cannot comprehend or explain in the world. Rituals can feel very comforting when navigating the acute challenges we face in the underworld.

When Inanna descends on the autumn equinox I build a dark altar, with a black cloth, to honour the Ereshkigal part of the year. And at the spring equinox I change the altar cloth to a white one and make a light altar to honour Inanna and the brighter seasons of the year.

If the time of year you are reading this book does not correlate with these seasons, you can choose to honour your internal seasons instead. There is no wrong way of doing this, so be creative and allow your altar to be a mirror for your inner life. Suggestions for things to put on your altar are:

- a candle

- statues

- photographs

- natural objects: flowers, feathers, shells or stones

- a drawing/painting/some other artwork

- a poem.

This list is far from exhaustive so be creative and follow your impulse.

DESCENT

RISING

Gate One
the crown – mind

Cycle completes

Gate Two
intuition – third eye

Feminine and masculine
enter new partnership

Gate Three
voice – throat

Geshtinanna offers
compassion

Gate Four
love – heart

Inanna reckons
with sacrifice and
desire for life

Gate Five
power – solar plexus

Sacrifices Dumuzi

Gate Six
sexuality – womb

Inanna finds
her "no"

Gate Seven
roots/belonging – vulva

Inanna rises flanked by
Galla demons

death

Transition
Enki's emissaries
offer empathy

Ereshkigal grants food
and water of life

THE DESCENT

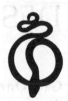

This is the place
where all the paths
you thought would bring you home
converge and fall away
and you must stand still
or step back
or step off
into an impossible wilderness
where the only voice
is your own voice
or there is no voice at all.
And the tide of habit draws you back
to the path that is already pressed in the void
that measures the dark
and feels like home
but now you are homeless
and crave the dark
out of whose black clay
words form
that have never been spoken
from flesh and breath
that is only yours.
There is no direction here
and none allowed
only the steady throb
of something wild and hungry
inside you
and the next breath.

from "Autobiography of 1994" by Kim Rosen

Gate One – The Mind

As Inanna enters the first gate, from her head her crown is taken.

To which Inanna asks, *"What is this?"*

The Gatekeeper replies,

"Quiet Inanna, the ways of the underworld are perfect, they may not be questioned."

At the first gate our crown is removed. On a personal level, it is our upper-world crown that is taken: the way we know ourselves and the way that others know us. This can include the roles we play in the world: mother, daughter, lover, wife and so forth. The crowns we wear may also include our profession: doctor, teacher, carer, writer… Inextricably linked to this, is the way that we think we are seen by others (whether that is imagined or real) and the way that we want to be seen by others. For example, we may be attached to being viewed as reliable, trustworthy, generous and so on. Most of us shape ourselves to a greater or lesser extent around these roles and personal attributes. Among them, there are parts of us we hope will be seen, and parts that, consciously and subconsciously, we try to hide. There is nothing wrong with this *per se,* but when we become strongly identified with being this way and not that way, our crown can become confining and restrictive. This perpetuates the spilt between Inanna and Ereshkigal. In this context, Inanna can be seen as our upperworld idealised self: the way we like to see ourselves and try to be seen. Ereshkigal is our shadow underworld self, the parts we try to hide or are ashamed of.

Journalling exercise

The purpose of this exercise is to get to know the Inanna and Ereshkigal parts of yourself a little better.

1. Make a list of all the ways you like to be seen by others. If you get stuck, think of specific people or roles in your life and write a list of how you like to be thought of by that person, or in that role.

---

2. Then make a list of all the ways you hope not to be seen by others. If you get stuck, include all the things you consider to be the worst attributes of humans in general and see what comes up.

Then read through your lists and notice which ones hold the most voltage for you. Underline one attribute from each and write about a specific real-life example of:

3. How you tried to be seen in a certain light – what did you do, say, wear etc. to promote your Inanna self?

4. How the thing that you so dislike lives in you? If you can discover it then ask – what tactics do you employ to avoid it? How do you hide your Ereshkigal attributes? What do you try not to do, say, wear, show about this part of yourself?

You may be able to feel, just from doing this exercise, how much of our energy is used to keep our crowns in place. We all do this on some level. From a young age, we receive messages from our family and society about what is valued and what is not. We can see this in our education system, whose focus is to get children through exams that assess academic intelligence, judged by a particular hierarchy of knowledge, rather than gardening the soul of each child as it starts to emerge. That is not to deny that there are many wonderful teachers in education. But I have seen, in my own schooling and that of my children, how much pressure there is for educational achievement to be quantifiable. Add to that other agents of socialisation, such as the family, religion, media, peer group and cultural ideals, and we can begin to form a picture of what and who have helped to shape our crowns. This shaping can mean that, sadly, many of us end up wearing a crown that we have not chosen, or one that is compromised by the pressures of our sociocultural structures and ideals. For example, the stifled creativity of the teacher, who cannot teach freely and responsively to the soul of the child.

A part of the heroine's journey is to become more and more of who we really are – to become more authentic and to heal the split inside of our selves. In her book, *Saved by a Poem*, poet and teacher Kim Rosen offers *two keys to authenticity*, that I feel are also key ingredients of the heroine's journey,

The first is a willingness to welcome feelings of being unseen, unheard and misunderstood. [...] Paradoxically, it is only when you are willing to be unseen that you can be truly visible. Without that willingness, some percentage of your life energy is always tied up in subconsciously trying to be seen as you'd like to be seen, and along with this, by necessity, you will probably be trying to protect yourself against judgment and rejection.

The second key is seemingly the opposite: a willingness to be seen, yet as you really are, including all sides of yourself, not just the ones you are proud of.

The Inanna aspect of us has an impulse to hide and cover up the Ereshkigal part to keep her crown intact. Rosen's keys help us to unlock the gates of our authentic expression, so that we can be all that we are. But, when we meet our shadow self, and particularly when we fear it might have been seen by others, our tendency is to quickly try to re-cover it. Have you ever had that nagging feeling after a night out, or after a sensitive conversation with another, where you feel a bit exposed and keep reworking it over in your mind? This replaying the scenario is how our idealised self tries to cover over what we fear has been exposed. What we are feeling is the compulsion in us to 'fix it' – to fix Ereshkigal. We spend so much of our life energy doing this, but our attempts to avoid the discomfort of any exposure can actually smother our authenticity and keeps our Inanna and Ereshkigal aspects estranged. In this way, our crown can become part of a mask that hides who we truly are.

Rosen goes on to reference Eve and Adam who, after biting into the apple from the Tree of Knowledge, become aware of their nakedness and experience shame for the first time. In response, they desperately try to cover themselves. As we descend we strip naked again. Contrary to the biblical teaching of Eve and Adam, Inanna becoming naked in the descent is actually a return to innocence. I relish that turn-around. But, the shame that arises when we meet our shadow aspects all too often makes us run for the fig leaf, or even some much heftier armour, to protect ourselves.

Journal prompt – an exercise to help us to meet Ereshkigal

1. Think of a time when you felt exposed or when you found yourself ruminating over something that happened. What happened and what did it feel like?

2. Breathe into that feeling and drop in the question: What part of myself was I afraid had been seen? What was I trying to cover?

3. What are my core fears around this part of me being exposed? Rejection, abandonment, being unlovable? There is usually a core fear that compels us to keep Ereshkigal in the dark.

4. Notice what happens in the body when you meet this part of yourself? How are you breathing? What contracts, what are the feelings that arise or numb out? Can you meet this part or does it feel too difficult or unknown?

5. To finish, make some notes on what you have noticed. Sometimes the feelings that arise as we start to meet Ereshkigal can be very strong. I always find it helps me massively to remember – *no feeling lasts forever.* If you feel overwhelmed I recommend seeking out some support.

Our mind, symbolised by our crown, likes to control and does not like to be told that *the ways of the underworld are perfect and may not be questioned.* This unequivocal reply is difficult for the mind to grasp. We would prefer a good reason or explanation to hang onto. But, in many circumstances, there is not an obvious explanation, perhaps ever. One of the most challenging things about life is that things are taken from us, people die and we get hurt and there isn't always a good reason. In the descent, we must come face to face with our losses and our own mortality. We might be fooled into thinking that the crowns we wear will help us to circumvent unhappiness or death. Subconsciously, we may think, *if I just do this, if I am just good enough, important enough, I will survive.* We all want immunity from suffering. But we are all mortal and no one is immune. There are many deaths that we have to face in one lifetime. Death is, to an extent, incomprehensible to the mind: both births and deaths are physical processes that we can only live our way to 'understanding'.

False crowns and waking up to the 'Good Daughter' within

Esoterically speaking, the crown chakra is also our doorway to spirit, the portal to our higher self and the gateway through which it is said the spirit leaves when we die. When we are wearing a false crown it can become a lid blocking our inspiration and our joy. Those wearing a false crown rarely feel their spirit lift and can easily become depressed by the weight of the crown. Many of the trappings of a 'successful life' that may give us a certain amount of security, can actually become the stagnant pools in which we can no longer thrive and grow. On the surface, we may have many things that we need, but something inside us is starving. For those of us who have been praised for our sharp mind and have made a decent living by it, having our crown removed is unthinkable. Furthermore, the workplace is still not designed for women to thrive, and the professional roles that women fill are frequently less well-paid. Therefore, for women to give up our work crown, a crown that has likely been hard-earned (even if it is a crown that we did not want or chose), is a huge risk.

Women have a hard time saying no because it feels so good to be chosen, especially by the king. We enjoy pleasing daddy, our boss, our co-worker, our lover. We don't want to disappoint others; so much of our self-image is invested in making other people happy. Our internal little girl doesn't want to be left behind. It's too painful to choose not to join the fun. And we need the income.

Maureen Murdock, *The Heroine's Journey*

Murdock's words make me squirm inside. To this day, so much of me still wants to reject them. Yet, as I descended, I had to face the fact that this truth lived inside of me. I was a feminist since my teens, my mum was a feminist and my dad was also pretty gender aware. But when I descended, I woke up to all the negative ways that patriarchy had still seeped into me. A painful and inevitable part of the descent is admitting how we have embodied patriarchal values to our own detriment and how they are woven into our familial and social systems, and inevitably, our crown. As a daughter of patriarchy, I had to admit to myself, that part of me was totally geared up in pursuit of the Father's love and approval (in all the ways that shows up in our lives) and all the ways that I had colluded with my own oppression, in order to be the 'chosen one' in his eyes.

As we descend, the 'good daughter' is an aspect of ourselves that has to die.

In order to compost the good daughter crown, we have to wake up to how much we value it, how it has influenced our choices, our relationships and our feelings about ourselves. Embodiment coach, Priscilla Rogers' story is a visceral example of composting the crown:

> "I was in my last year of grad school and I was binge-watching an interview series called 'The Good Life Project'. I realized I'd been hoodwinking myself into thinking I could play both sides, that I could fit into the social order game and live a good enough life for my soul to bear. I knew I didn't want to get my PhD anymore – the path my parents paved for me. The path that would give me social clout, relief from my blackness, a seat at the table. I would fit in. A Masters seemed like a bargain.
>
> But one day I found myself on the floor of my Harlem apartment sobbing deep guttural cries of grief and emotional turmoil. I was in my last semester at NYU and I realised I'd bought into the colonial white supremacist and patriarchal systems of abuse. That my creativity was being stamped out and crushed. I was being taught to hate myself, my hair, my body, my skin colour and my femininity. It all came crashing down in me in that singular moment, as I writhed in emotional pain on the floor. I have been in reclamation mode ever since. Reclaiming the shamed and lost parts of me. Reconnecting with my creative pleasure and power. And most recently connecting to my body and most sensuous self. I am sure that each part we call back home is a political act of power. As Audre Lorde says, 'Revolution is not a one-time event'."

As Priscilla names so clearly, she had bought into upperworld ideals. In Western culture, these include whiteness, maleness, academia, body ideals, respectability and more. We shape our bodies and crowns to fit in, but at what cost? When our crown is taken, we must give up a lot of what we think we know about ourselves, what we think we are and are supposed to be. As we descend what we are likely to discover is that:

Some of our closest personal relationships are enmeshed in our false crowns.

This is what makes us want to hold onto our crowns so tightly. We don't want to disrupt the family system, relationships, workplace, or community. But when the incongruence inside us becomes as deathly as the risk of sacrificing our crowns, we finally submit, like Inanna does as she strips back to her bare, naked self.

Composting the crown

We have to compost what we were to give mulch for the descent, mulch that nourishes our roots. But, as Priscilla describes, the loss of the illusion is painful, firstly, because it means losing our perceived place in the world. But also because it can be deeply disturbing to wake up to all that we have not previously been able to see. In my experience, it shakes our sense of knowing to its core.

Composting the crown can also be threatening to those around us and the changes taking place in us are often felt by significant others in our lives who might say, *"you are not who I thought you were"* or *"have you lost your mind?"* In a sense, we have lost our minds, in a good way: we have lost the part of our mind that is willing to collude with the dominator and the oppression that we have internalised. We have lost the capacity to morph ourselves into a new good daughter shape. If we have become a part of others' identities, then as we die, part of them also dies. People find it hard to endure the composting of our crown, because the vast majority of us are collectively geared towards wanting the loving gaze of the strong Father. Stepping out of the kingdom takes courage and not many people want to go there. To some, it brings intolerable discomfort and, as a result, we may be rejected by the people who we thought loved us the most. As Linda Hartley states,

> We are reminded that in death, all are equal, and all must be humbled by death, stripped naked of our achievements and power in the upperworld, for they have no place in this realm.

This *all are equal* notion that Hartley refers to is a threat to the in-built structural inequality through which our dominator society exists. Therefore, to give up our crown is a radical act of rebellion against the way of things. However, even if we are absolutely dedicated to the composting of the crown, it is still immensely destabilising. If we give up a *good* job, leave a *good* marriage, no longer attend the *good* church and so on, we step outside of a kind of belonging. This gate challenges our rational choices and asks us to follow the thread of soul which leads us into the dark and does not offer a clear Promised Land. It asks us to slow down, yield and re-commune with our true nature, through which we begin to encounter aspects of ourselves, and the world that we have previously been blind to.

We often set off on our heroines' journeys on a path of reclamation, not knowing that Ereshkigal will strip us bare before we get the chance to reclaim anything. As the tangible physicality of Priscilla's words name, we have to admit and grieve what has been hurt, lost and ignored first. We have to feel our shame, rage and pain, in order to feel how deeply what we have colluded with is embodied in us. These are not just ideas. When we compost the crown, we begin to feel the truth of this. The good news is, that as we admit all of the difficult feelings, we also open the door to the possibility of pleasure and sensuality as well. Even the most challenging feelings we experience can, with time, be a portal to our greatest aliveness.

The heroine's journey is an erotic initiation that returns us to our sensual nature: our *eros*. Capitalist patriarchy prizes *logos* – the principles of reason and judgement – over *eros*. The rational, scientific mind provides us with something we can measure, that can be converted into monetary gain or power, through which we are encouraged to dominate other people, ideas, places and the body. Whereas, when our crowns are taken, we begin to *feel* our connectedness and realise that everything we have is borrowed, from our roles, our home, even the body we call our own. One day, all of this will be composted back into the whole. Our mind is so keen to put us in the centre of everything, to create a legacy. But erotic soul life is a remembering that our human stories are just one part of much bigger picture. When asked what the old stories are crying out to tell us mythologist and author, Sharon Blackie suggests,

> *That sense that we are a part of the Earth's story, the Land's story, that we are not always the heroes or protagonists of the story, that we are just a part of it…that the story is often rarely about us.*

Historically, it seems we did used to have more sense of this. According to Blackie, right up to the sixteenth century in Irish tradition, the crowning of the king would have been accompanied by a ceremony to marry the land. The king entered partnership with the Earth and in this way was seen as a custodian of the land. It was understood that if the king had bad judgement, that the land too would suffer and become a wasteland. In this marriage he pledged to be a protector of the land, but was also answerable to the land.

In modern times, this sense of partnership has been eroded and individualism is rife. Having lived in a dominator model for so many years, winning and losing, doing better than others, is something we are encouraged to strive for, so when we 'fail' it can feel like death. But actually, mistakes are probably our greatest gifts. Through our mistakes, we breed humility and through humility, we cultivate connection. We only fall as far as the floor, then we learn that the floor is the thing that helps us get back up. In the face of the devastation of our planet, this falling down onto the Earth seems essential. In her book, *Eastern Body, Western Mind*, Anodea Judith elucidates,

The crown chakra is the thousand petalled lotus. Most people think of the petals
as reaching up into the heavens; actually, the lotus petals turn downward like
a sunflower, dripping nectar into the crown and down through the chakras.

I love this image. The lotus roots in muck, down into the fecund dirt of the Earth. So too do our roots need to come back down into the mud. The heroine's journey is the path of downward mobility. This downward growth requires us to yield to the mystery and humble ourselves. Dying and birthing are messy, holy rites of passage. As the crown dissolves we enter our humanness and submit to the unknown, not only on a personal level, but a collective level. Collectively, we have forgotten how to live in partnership with Her, it is my hope that it is not too late for us to remember. I believe that our personal descents are a part of our collective waking up.

Paradoxically, it is only through the recognition of all that
we do not know, that we can truly open to the question: who
am I and what am I supposed to do with my life?

Gate Two – The Third Eye

When she entered the second gate, the small lapis beads were taken from Inanna's neck.

Lapis lazuli is one of the world's most sought-after stones and is associated with the third eye. The third eye can be thought of as the centre of our knowledge, the kind of knowing that reaches beyond the cognitive mind, often referred to as our intuitive centre. Our eyes, placed on the right and left sides of the body, work in tandem to give us the full picture, but inevitably we still have a tendency to think dualistically. The third eye is the site of our central vision, the place where we are not pulled in one direction or the other. From this wisdom, we can enter into equanimity and perception beyond 'this or that'. It is also a portal to our spirituality, higher consciousness and a sense of the beyond.

Historically, the most intuitive women are the ones who have suffered the most. They were the 'witches' who were burned at the stake. Even to this day, women who follow their instinctive knowing and speak out from their own authority will often be heavily criticised for having a voice. Women are regularly attacked on social media, receive death threats and are 'put in their place' by the violence of a world that still wants to keep women down.

In England, burning was the most common punishment for women for many crimes against patriarchy. It matters. It does. Because those flames that burned our foremothers in their hundreds of thousands burn us still today, albeit metaphorically, for exactly the same reason.
A woman lived under threat of being burned alive for living, speaking or acting in any way which contradicted or questioned the cultural norms which surrounded her: medical, spiritual or hierarchical.

Lucy H. Pearce, *Burning Woman*

Often when we speak about the third eye, we section off the head from the body. The notion of transcending the physical body, moving up into the higher centres of awareness, is the goal of many spiritual traditions and practices. However, in contemporary culture, so many of us are already 'walking heads', so mind-focused and dissociated that we do not adequately listen to the body. So, I question: how healthy is it that our spiritual lives perpetuate these patterns?

In my view, spiritual practices should both support and challenge our ways of being to help us to grow and mature. Monotheistic religions cite God, as being 'above' in heaven. The kingdom of heaven being above the Earth, not of the Earth. Collectively, secular narratives also constantly seek to elevate humans above the Earth, above the animal, to the rational. In the dominator paradigm, we see animals as primitive or less than, because of our big brains. But look where our big brains are taking us: headlong into our own self destruction. For me, heaven and hell are alive and well, right now, here on Earth. Every time I see a bee hovering on a flower, or the spiral of a fern, I am witnessing a miracle. I know myself to be part of a fragile, alive, intricate, mysterious system more complex than I can possibly cognise, but my third eye can feel it – I can feel it. Who teaches the geese to migrate, who teaches us to birth, who teaches the seasons to change? I believe this 'knowing' is the same energy as the energy of our intuition. If I acknowledge this, I re-enter the truth that 'my' intuition is not only 'mine', it is actually part of my divine animal instinct. An instinct that is part of my Earth connection, part of the web of life, of which I am just one part. Therefore, I believe intuition is not just *our* intuition, it is ancient and inextricably linked to the magic of the natural world around us, the mycelium of which we are an integral part. But because of the painful dissociative patterns in our bodies, we often separate from this truth.

Trauma and intuition

Trauma and wounding can freeze part of our aliveness in the past. When animals in the wild experience trauma they shake, which discharges the energy of the trauma. This is believed to be the reason why animals in the wild do not experience PTSD, but animals in captivity, and humans, do. Oftentimes we are not in a situation where we get to shake off and discharge. Consequently, the energy of the experience gets lodged in our systems, as mentioned earlier, like a scratch in a record. Though the scratch happened in the past, the stuckness of the pattern replays in present time and shapes how we cope with life. For this reason, I don't feel we can have a conversation about intuition without a conversation about trauma.

For many years, I worked at a counselling service for women who had survived sexual trauma and abuse. I held a space where the women could do yoga-based movement to begin to feel and befriend their bodies again. When the body feels like an unsafe space, doing some simple, conscious movement can be a way of contacting and beginning to trust our somatic experience again. Many of the women who came to my sessions rarely left home. Their intuition told them that the world wasn't safe and so they would avoid going out. Was this true? Well, the world is not safe, we are mortal and we know there is danger. But we are likely to be safe enough going to the shop in broad daylight, or out to pick our children up from school. These women had had their sense of safety eroded at such a young age, that their bodies, and therefore the body of the world, did not feel safe. This is an acute example of how our intuition can be shaped by trauma at a core level. What we are intuiting becomes directed by what happened in the past, rather than what is here and now. Of course, our past experiences can help us discern what is likely to happen now, and if we have suffered abuse, then we do what we can to survive and live a life that we can endure. What I am pointing to in this example is that intuition is not as simple as we might initially think. Intuition and our nervous systems' responses are affected and coloured by our past experiences.

The first time I dissociated from my body was when I was born. My birth was traumatic for both me and my mum. I was pulled out by my head in a forceps delivery. Years later, having traced it back somatically through breathwork and therapy, I believe this created a dissociative pattern which has played and replayed in my life. My mum has always been incredibly intuitive, she has also always had a long menstrual cycle and intuitively felt that I wasn't ready to be born. But the medical system overrode her intuition and forced induction onto her body and mine, resulting in high blood pressure, an epidural and a forceps delivery. Of course, we rarely think about the impact of our birth experience, and it was only years later, when doing an antenatal yoga teacher training, that some of my implicit memories came to light. We were in circle, speaking about hospital births and as I began to speak this uncontrollable rage and emotion came out through my voice and body. I couldn't hold back the tears, which was such a surprise to me, as I had no idea that I was even carrying this pain and anger.

Having worked with many women who have suffered birth trauma, I feel that our approach to birth is, to an extent, modelled on the dominator dynamic: some medical professionals exert power over a birthing woman's body when she is most vulnerable, rather than being guided by her. They may do this with the best of intentions, but our upperworld medical systems are sometimes very disconnected and mistrusting of the sacred, innate process of birth which, as we looked at earlier, goes right back to the root of patriarchal medicine.

Birth is one of the most potent examples of deeply embodied feminine intuition. It is a process that expands, opens the gates of our body and invites us to go way beyond anything we could imagine and yet towards something that we inherently know. Birth is here, happening now, and it is as ancient as time. This does not mean that all births will be straightforward, or that women aren't intuiting well enough if they cannot birth vaginally. Sometimes, complications happen. Life happens. So why am I speaking about birth when speaking about the third eye? Because the energy of the deep feminine, unequivocally embodied in the birthing process, tells us that intuition is about the body, not only the mind. For me, birth is one of the best examples of a human, intuitive, animal process. I believe that our Western attitude towards birth speaks volumes about our distorted relationship with the power held in feminine intuitive processes.

One of the costs of my dissociative pattern, combined with socialisation that taught me to overly accommodate others, is that a sense of my own boundaries did not come easily to me. When we are dissociated we cannot feel our bodies, we cannot hear what we are a "yes" to and what we are a "no" to. I notice this can be more prevalent in clients who have had church-based upbringings with heavy socialisation around being 'good'. Whatever religion or culture we have been raised in helps shape our expectations, and what we think we should or can expect.

Cultural rules, expectations and the misshaping of ourselves

Fiza Noor's story is an example of this,

"My first descent would have been when I came to the UK. I think that was the first time of feeling like an 'other' and was where I learned to edit, adapt and assimilate. There was a fight, of Western versus traditional culture, that made me feel that I was living two completely different lives, in different parts of my existence. There are aspects of both cultures that I can completely align myself with, and there are aspects of those cultures that I completely reject.

My second descent would probably be when I got married. It was an arranged marriage, but I don't think the marriage was a problem: I went in with my full consent. But I loved his family more than I loved the man. The first descent was about who I want to be, and who I am forced to be. The second descent was more about what I want, and how I recognise what I want. I started to have to question how I know what I want, versus what others want for me – differentiating those two… There is only so much you can do for others, then there's a point when you have to start learning and living for yourself.

I was in my early twenties when I got divorced, I was in my final year at university. There were family crises, my dad was really unwell, he had cancer and there were numerous emotions and things going on. Then I qualified as a midwife and just as I thought I was reaching the end of the tunnel and scraping my way back up, I had a major car accident and almost died. I went to almost a literal otherworld. I was pretty unconscious, doped up and out of it. I lost a stone in a month. I had to learn how to walk again. I had to pay attention to being, in a very literal sense.

The concept of healing is very different in different cultures. In my culture, if someone is sick, you all live it: everyone in the family visits them, and gives them their prayers and blessings. But having grown up in this dual world, whereas my mum was very comfortable with people visiting me, I was not. My bed was in the living room, downstairs, and I would wake up and someone would be there, and my mum would be showing me to them. And that's just doing what's culturally acceptable, in our culture. But, it's not realising the boundaries and the needs of your child. Because they [my parents] never had that boundary set for them. I didn't realise that there were boundaries until very recently, because for me, boundaries had always been blurred. Expectations in one part of my life were completely different in another part of my life. And because of the ever-rotating concepts of cultural rules and expectations, I was constantly trying to fix myself. You know the square peg in a round hole analogy? I was chipping away at my corners, sanding them down so I could fit into this circle. I was trying to be whole, but actually I was hollow."

I feel that Fiza's descent gives a very clear example of the way that culture shapes us. This also affects our relationship with our intuition. Many times we are actively socialised to override our intuitive responses in order to be polite or to accommodate cultural norms, even if they are in conflict with our instincts. What I hear in Fiza's story is that the two cultures shone a light on each other and, in the end, gave her a portal through which to question: what are *my* boundaries? What are *my* needs? Fiza continues,

"For a long time, I never really focused on myself, I was too busy focusing on the world, fitting in and focusing on the family and their expectations, and their needs. One day, on the bed, I had a realization that I had almost died. I had been saving money, but I thought, what am I going to do with that money? Because when you're from a socio-economically deprived background, you are always unsure about money and having the back-up of savings is really important. But my priorities changed. I wanted to have experiences of life which had been limited to me earlier because of culture and expectations. I was an adult divorced woman, with means of my own, I could make different choices. I had a realisation that if I don't get up now, I will never get up. That was my changing point."

Meeting Ereshkigal in her near-death experience activated a new authority within Fiza, and, as she hung on the hook in the living room of her family home, she began to awaken to her own desires, and the urge to follow them.

Sacrificing dogma – coming home to our intuitive nature and spirit

When Inanna's lapis beads are removed, the veil lifts on the upperworld dogma that she has absorbed. In patriarchy this dogma is mostly created and held in place by the Sky Gods and the elevated masculine, embodied in the myth by

Dumuzi. By sacrificing the dogma, she can enter into new relationship with her true spiritual nature and her embodied intuitive self. As Fiza explains, her own longings and needs were buried under layers of cultural and familial expectation. As we travel down through the gates of the underworld, this starts to shift. During this process, we contact any unprocessed trauma and grief that has had to be buried in order to conform to the world as we have known it.

> "The first thing I did was say: I am going back to work. At this point, I had a midwifery job and five months post-accident I went back to work and continued with what I thought was healing. But actually I was just surviving. I became a workaholic, I worked as much as possible. For me, until early adulthood, I was going to be a wife and a mother and they were my expectations from my culture. If I couldn't be that, I decided I would be the best I could in the work I was doing."

What Fiza describes so eloquently is how she was flanked by the *galla* demons as she began to come back to life. They require a sacrifice and unless we are willing to make one, we will be haunted by our demons. Even though Fiza had started to try to put her own needs first, she had replaced her familial expectations with similar self-expectations *to be the best* at work. This is an internalisation of the elevated inner masculine that we must sacrifice as we rise. When our inner masculine and feminine are in this dynamic, the inner masculine becomes combative, perfectionist and domineering – nothing is ever enough. He becomes our inner dominator that keeps the good daughter in cycles of depletion. This might allow us to survive, but it isn't how we thrive.

Fiza's story is a great example of how the scripts that we have introjected drive us. These old scripts need to be brought to consciousness and transformed. The good daughter says, *"I am worthless unless..."* or *"I am not enough"* and the elevated dominant inner masculine backs this up with, *"You must work harder"*, *"That's not good enough"*. Their dialogue creates a toxic dynamic that drives us to overwork and prevents us rising. In this purgatory, we lose true connection to life. As Fiza names,

> "In my midwifery job, I was seeing things that were not okay, but

up until this point, I had been silent, and silence is compliance. I was getting frustrated with myself and others. I was seeing an unjust world, I was seeing racial biases, abuse, poor outcomes… I was seeing double standards. I was just not happy with what I was seeing. At this time, I went for an interview and for the first time, I challenged the panel. I got the job, after which they gave me free reign to write my own job title, my own description. For the first time, I wasn't put in a structure that I had to fit in, I was given the space to grow and evolve. I didn't realise how suffocated I had felt until this opportunity. Before that, I was working all hours and I wasn't sleeping because I was so angry at everything I was seeing. And I had really big issues around hierarchy. Traditionally, I was taught to submit to hierarchy. It's an intergenerational trauma, that is often taught in ethnic minority communities, especially the communities from the South Asian continent that suffered from the partition. It's a coping mechanism, a way to survive: a lesson our parents learnt and taught us, thinking they were teaching us how to survive, not realising that we now have the privilege and capacity to thrive. So, over time, I went from being obedient to hierarchy, to challenging hierarchy, in a professional respectful manner, but in doing so, I ended up raising my head above the parapet."

The intergenerational trauma that Fiza names is significant and brings even more gravitas to the domination and oppression playing out within her. We can be carrying trauma from our ancestral wounding that we do not even know about. The descent helps us uncover it. When Fiza, *stuck her head above the parapet,* she made a sacrifice. She started to risk being seen and heard, and challenged the hierarchy that she had been so conditioned to accept. In trusting and reconnecting with her intuition and desire, she sacrificed the elevated masculine and freed herself to rise, thereby changing the shape of her story.

Embodied intuition

At the second gate, Inanna enters a sense of spiritual and cultural homelessness, where she discovers what is holding her beneath human structures and expectations.

Fiza spoke to how her work as a midwife has supported her heroine's journey,

"In my religion, the belief is that when a woman is in labour, or a person is in the throes of birth, they are the closest to God that they can ever be. There are two ways of looking at that. One, that they are closest to God because they are bringing birth, they are bringing life to the world, as God did. Or they are so close to death, that they are close to God. So, people often think of birth as a beautiful experience, which it is. But you also see the most horrific things happen in these times. When I say horrific, I mean loss. Loss of a whole life, a whole family that could have been. You see all the emotions that come with all the triggers that the whole person brings into that birth room. You hear terrible things around abuse, rape, violence… You witness a person go through a journey in their own body for the first time, that they have never experienced before. Or even if it's a subsequent time, that they have never experienced before. You see how they face and overcome and continue to move on. There are so many lessons to be learnt in that birth room.

This work has held the keys to me, accepting me as I am. Because, in accepting all those individuals that came to me for care, I began to realise that I could be an individual too. Because if I can accept others that I care for in this way, then I can respect myself enough to care for myself in this way."

When we birth, we meet Ereshkigal, and midwives are the Ninshuburs of those births. As a midwife, you witness the descent and, as Fiza describes, the whole spectrum of humanness you might encounter there. Many of our dominant Western cultural narratives focus on mind over matter. Birth is the opposite of that: it is an embodied, all-encompassing process and so too are our heroines' journeys. In this respect, birth is the perfect metaphor for the spiritual path of

Exercise to support embodied intuition

This is a simple exercise that can support our embodied intuition. When we over identify with others, or are rushing, it's much harder to feel intuitively. When we rush we tend to be energetically ahead of ourselves. And when we have gone towards the other, we often sit forwards in our seat, or over-give in some way. When we do this a lot, it can disconnect us from ourselves and our intuition. The simple action of sitting back in our seat, can be a somatic reminder to come back to ourselves that changes the energy in our bodies. Try it out in day-to-day situations, when you catch yourself sitting forwards, consciously sit back and notice what shifts.

You can also play with this whilst walking. Find a space where you can walk across the room. Place your fingers on your third eye (between your eyebrows). Then walk being lead from your third eye, let it pull your body forwards as you walk and notice how you feel. How do your feet connect to the floor, how steady do you feel, how connected to the rest of your body, how does your energy system respond?

Then stop, and take a breath.

Now place your finger tips on the back of your head, behind your third eye and walk from there. Again, notice the effect, how you feel, how connected you are to the rest of your body, how do your feet connect to the floor now, how does your energy system respond?

Pause and take a breath. Notice what you observe.

When we have awareness of the back body it changes our relationship to the world. It means we 'have our own backs'. This is a simple way to somatically invite the front body (what we can see) and the back body (what is out of view) into a new relationship. Some people may find they sit back a lot and need to come forwards into life, that's good information too. Really there is no right or wrong. It's more about tapping into our felt sense, that helps us access our deeper knowing.

the feminine. Ereshkigal is so important for our spiritual practice because she represents the dark of our embodied humanity. She holds all the parts of ourselves that we go to great lengths to hide or avoid: the parts that we are ashamed of, the parts of us that we fear will destroy us (or those we love) and the parts that are suffering. We may think we need to work harder to transcend her, but actually we need to include and learn from her.

Giving birth to my daughters was one of the catalysts for my own descent. In my heroine's journey, I experienced some of the most elevating, evocative, transcendent experiences of my life, coupled with some of the worst pain, darkness and heartbreak. The gate of my third eye only really opened up when all the centres below it could support the experience. And the lower centres of my body could only support the experience when they were earthed and rooted in my human mulch, not because I had transcended my humanness.

Like a lotus flower, I blossomed most radiantly
through a deepened rooting in the muck.

Gate Three – The Throat

The patterns of your life
repeat themselves until you listen.
Forgive this. Say now
what you have to say.

from "The Art of Fugue: VI" by Jan Zwicky

When she enters the third gate, Inanna's double strand of beads is taken from her.

The beads are symbolic of Inanna's voice and expression. Our voice is one of our central instruments of communication and, as such, has so many layers of our experience held within it. Layers that have been shaped by our conditioning, upbringing and habitual ways of being. Have you ever noticed how some people only speak from their neck upwards? Or that others make you feel tense when they speak? Whilst others may sound like a cello, full and woody.

I had never really thought about my voice much until I discovered poetry.

I remember the first time my therapist read a poem to me, it touched me in a way that I had not felt before. It's no exaggeration to say that this experience reshaped the course of my life and work. But when I began to speak poetry myself, I felt like there was a veneer between my feelings and my voice, a tangible disconnect between what I felt and the freedom to express it. It was as though the feelings were in the underworld and I could not imagine how to possibly reveal the true depths hidden there. But I longed to.

The inflections and textures learned in childhood are reinforced over and over by repetition. Your voice moves through your growing body like a river carving its path through earth. All of your musculature grows around these habits of sound. [...] Your body falls into habitual patterns of speaking, leaving behind many possibilities of sound and feeling.

Kim Rosen, *Saved by a Poem*

What I noticed was that my voice could not be forced out, because the more I tried, the more evasive the submerged layers seemed to be. Like the heroine's journey, the process of revealing the lost colours of my expression could not be done by will. It required curiosity, play, vulnerability and surrender to *all* of my feelings. What we do and don't say has the power to shape our lives. How we communicate what's true for us (or not) can create patterns of experience that repeat again and again *until we listen,* as Zwicky's beautiful poem elucidates. At this gate Inanna opens to her lost voices and gets to feel, like I did, how she is estranged from them.

As part of his work on Polyvagal Theory, Stephen Porges researched the role of the voice in regulating and toning our vagus nerve. In female bodies, the vagus nerve connects from the brain and innervates the throat, voice box, heart, diaphragm, gut and cervix. Studies have shown that sounding actually tones the vagus nerve. When I say tone, I don't mean it as we often think of it, like a hard abdominal six pack. I am referring to tone as our capacity to be responsive. For example, in optimum tone, a muscle should be able to activate when needed and then be able to return to a place of rest with relative ease. A well-toned nervous system is the same. Ideally it is responsive when we need to activate, or if we are under threat, and can relax when we are not. To have the right to speak and be heard is an important part of being in the world. When we feel heard, we feel recognised and valued. Whereas if we are continually not heard, or have negative experiences around our voice, this affects our nervous system. As Porges names, "The speaking, the listening, this dynamic action, is really our pathway into shared experiences and connecting with another." Amongst other things Porges' theory explores how as humans we co-regulate one another through our shared communication.

I am so moved by the power of the voice and have beheld many people as they have reclaimed their lost voices. With practice and time, we can reconfigure the patterning of our responses and move beyond our habitual ways of speaking and sounding to whole new landscapes of expression.

Jo's experience is a powerful illustration of this. Jo came to work with me in the Butterfly Mystery School. In the past she had experienced domestic abuse and was suffering with the lasting effects of PTSD. Butterfly includes movement, breathwork and sounding practices that encourage spontaneous expression. When we begin to work in this way it can sift any underlying wounding or trauma to the surface. In the first year, if anyone made a loud sound in the room, Jo would have to leave, as her flight response was activated. Her body had such an ingrained association with loud voices being a violent threat, that it would activate an involuntary trauma response in Jo's body that told her that she was in danger and needed to escape. This also prohibited her own voice, in that she could not let out a loud shriek or shout, instead it would come out as shorter staccato sounds, or not at all. At first Jo wasn't sure that she would be able to be in the room, or continue with the course. But with support, she decided she wanted to try and work with it.

> "Over time I became more at ease with loud sounds as they became more expected. Eventually, they could even prompt a smile, as both they and I fitted into the space. Though I did still have a flight reaction to unexpected sound, the work in Butterfly did help teach me to down-regulate."

Down-regulation refers to the ways that we can re-ground and calm a hyper-aroused nervous system. With PTSD our flight and fight responses tend to be hyper-sensitised, meaning they will kick in even when we are not in danger. This can be really exhausting and debilitating for the person suffering it and can make even benign environments feel very overwhelming and unsafe. To help facilitate Jo I suggested that when her flight response was triggered, she could actively look around the room to relocate herself in the here and now, whilst taking deep breaths to help her calm her nervous system. The seemingly simple act of moving our head and eyes to take in our environment can help us to relocate into the present moment. She also knew she could leave the room, with the presence and support of an assistant if she needed to, until she felt safe enough to re-enter the space. Gradually, she learned to use this simple technique to help down-regulate herself.

At the end of the second year an amazing shift occurred. She shared in the circle,

"I was at home last week and a door unexpectedly slammed and I screamed. Not short staccato sounds, but a loud continuous, spontaneous yelp."

I remember tears welling up in my eyes as she told me, because I recognised that the energy of Jo's own voice had on some level been allowed to fly free again. Jo shares,

"I did not completely lose inhibition sounding in the group, but over time this lowered. I felt more comfortable to give voice when the sounds around me were very loud, so my voice blended in."

I found this last statement really interesting, in that where loud sound had previously been very activating for Jo, later, loud sounds actually became supportive to her expressing sounds that were trapped and needed release.

Liberating our voice and expression

I first discovered the cervix-throat connection somatically in my own body, before I encountered Porges' work. I was in Ireland on retreat with Kim Rosen, who leads immersions in poetry, breathwork and self-enquiry that offered me a potent space for liberating feelings and expression. Nearby was a lake, which many women would go for walks around. I, too, went for walks, but all the while my antennae would be up for male predators. This hyper-vigilance for male predatory energy has been very pronounced in me and I would often wonder how my friends could so easily go for walks in the countryside or woods alone and not feel it, or at least not to the same degree as I did.

I had been exploring this fear pattern consciously as part of the retreat. One lunchtime, I did the lake walk whilst confronting this feeling of fear in myself. Afterwards we entered a session of movement to loud music that took me into a mini descent. I wailed, sounded, screamed and moaned my way through the layers of fear, out of the mind into the underworld of my body and all that was held around this deep oppression and tension inside. Eventually, I ended up kneeling with my vulva on the floor sounding from my pelvic bowl. I could feel my cervix vibrating, orgasmically pulsing through and moving the sounds that were spontaneously coming out of my mouth. I was completely inside and allowing the sound out, but out from the Earth, through cervix to mouth. The cervix, voice and whole canal of my body were freed in the tremors of my sounding. It was a deeply healing experience. The old fear of this predatory energy was on some level liberated and recapitulated by this experience and my relationship to walking alone has changed since. I would like to note here that it is not all on women to free ourselves. Whilst violence against women is such an accepted part of our culture, women will never feel free. But we can meet the trauma and stuckness in our bodies that we have internalised in response to this, and, in my experience, this can help us to feel more empowered and assertive.

It was months later, that I came across Olivia Bryant's online platform Self:Cervix, and through it Porges' work, where the scientific dots joined with my experience. My experience was a somatic teaching to me, about the cervix-voice connection. Though I didn't know anything about the vagus nerve at that time, my body had its own wisdom and this, not my mind, was what freed me.

The oppression of women's voices

Historically, the female voice has been marginalised, and to this day women who have a voice are often abused, trolled and heavily criticised in the public domain, in a way that men are not. In her book, *Women and Power – A Manifesto,* Mary Beard goes back 3,000 years to the start of Homer's Odyssey. She observes, "as Homer has it, an integral part of growing up, as a man, is learning to take control of public utterance and to silence the female of the species." Beard paints an in-depth picture of how society has formed ideas around which voices hold authority or *muthos* (men and often white able-bodied men) in public space and which don't (anyone who isn't a white man). This is one of the subconscious codes of our Western culture, which at best means that women have to try to adapt to be heard and, at worst, means women's voices are still woefully under-represented in the public sphere. There is still an oppressive misogynistic culture of harassment, threat and abuse on social media platforms such as Twitter, that tries to silence any woman who speaks out. As Beard highlights,

Those who do manage successfully to get their voice across often have to adopt some version of the 'androgyne' route. [...] That was what Margaret Thatcher* did when she took voice training specifically to lower her voice, to add the tone of authority that her advisors thought her high pitch lacked.

This is a prime example of how we have to adapt to the upperworld and may end up sacrificing our true natural expression to do so. I am focussing on female experience in a male world here, however, I acknowledge this issue does not only affect women, and that others who do not fit into our narrow structures of white wealthy masculinity also experience cultural oppression around the voice.

This is prohibitive to women stepping into their authority in work, personal relationships and in the embodiment of their own unique voice. A society that prioritises male voices in leadership, also undervalues female voices in those spaces. Women tend to be taken less seriously and in order to hold *muthos* must adapt ourselves to be very composed, unemotional and express ourselves in a tone more akin to a traditional male voice. But this is changing. I remember watching Laura Bates' excellent TED Talk on "Everyday Sexism". There was this woman, speaking such powerful words but in a very softly spoken, lyrical voice. I was captivated by her. This did not diminish her. In fact, for me, it had the opposite effect – I was inspired. It's so refreshing to me when people allow emotional expression as a part of their leadership. It brings empathy, heart and resonance to our voices that we cannot get in the more polished, traditional style of political rhetoric.

Nevertheless, I have found it quite frightening to step into a more feminine form of leadership: it is a vulnerable thing to forage off the beaten track and stand for something different. As we have already named, the burning of witches is not all that long ago and the fear that closes our throats is not rooted in nothing. It is rooted in a history of silencing, persecution and trauma that has taught us that to liberate our voices, is to risk being visible, in a society where visible women are hurt and attacked.

---

* The first female British Prime Minister.

*Whatever expression is not allowed, is not vanquished, it is
sent down into the underworld where it stays in exile.*

Reclaiming our lost voices

We may be mistaken in accepting that our current spectrum of expression is all
we have. But every time we speak in opposition to our truth, it is registered by
the body. Take a reasonably common example: we are super-busy and someone
asks us a favour, we should reasonably say *no,* but we find ourselves saying *yes.*
Or when we are really angry and instead of expressing it, we keep a mask on
our face and use a voice that is calm and collected. When we habitually mask or
negate our true feelings, we create tension in the body. The disconnect between
what we feel and what we show does not go unnoticed. Sometimes this capacity
to not show all of our feelings in the moment is useful. But when we have subconsciously entered a pattern of always overriding our true response to accommodate others, we are exiling a vital part of our expression. When Inanna's double strand of beads is taken, she enters a process of composting the voices that
were not hers and welcoming the voices that she has not yet met inside herself.
When we descend, we start to listen to what has not been said, all the voices and
sounds that have not been allowed, admitted or possibly even felt. Until now.

Kimberly Ann Johnson suggests that when women heal through down-regulat-
ing our nervous systems, we can feel more, before regaining the capacity to up-regulate back into healthy aggression (we explore this further in Chapter Nine). This
really resonates with the heroine's journey in that, first we descend back down into
the body and meet what has been hidden in our subconscious and implicit memory. And in the ascent, as we rise back into the world, we come into a more activated
state. A healthy nervous system is able to be responsive to any given situation,
from totally relaxed to highly activated and anything in between. In the heroine's
journey, we begin to bump into the parts of ourselves that are less known in this
spectrum of nervous system response. We can remember, reconnect and reclaim
our lost notes of expression and with it tone our nervous systems.

When Ereshkigal impales Inanna, she shows a pure expression of rage. Rage
tends to be more suppressed in women, partly because we are socialised to be
pleasing and accommodating, but also because if we are threatened by someone

bigger than us we instinctively fear that we may not survive a fight. This can mean that we mute all of our more assertive voices, and especially our rage. But if we can reclaim the wisdom held in Ereshkigal's wild rage it can serve a new voice.

The voice of "no".

What I have experienced in working with people who have experienced trauma, especially at the hands of a very aggressive parent or partner, is that part of the trauma response can be to submerge their own anger. Like in Jo's story, the fear of the other's rage manifests as a fear of our own. But anger itself is not bad. If we can reclaim our anger, we reclaim a part of our vital energy and, paradoxically, rather than making us more vulnerable, we will probably learn to protect and stand up for ourselves better.

Conversely, if we have relied on fight to get through life, our angry voice might be our most well-known voice. If this is you, discovering the more vulnerable, soft tones of your lost voices might be a new edge. At this gate we are led to ask: what needs to be said? What are the lost notes of our voices?

How can we welcome and embody the whole ensemble of voices within us?

Exploring your voice

This is an exercise I first experienced with Kim Rosen, that I now use with others.

1. First choose a poem or song.

2. Record yourself speaking the poem and listen back. Take some time to journal about what you hear and feel. What do you notice about your voice? Where does your breath sit inside your voice? What do you feel as you listen to your voice?

3. What, if anything, do you love about your voice? What, if anything, do you dislike about your voice? Is there anything else that you notice?

---

4. Write an autobiography of your voice. Think back through your life, from childhood to now, from the perspective of your voice's life story. What are key moments that you remember? Are there specific moments when you remember your voice being welcomed? Or denied? Are there specific people who encourage your voice, or conversely, people with whom you struggle to speak? Any key memories of experiences involving your voice, at school, at work, at home?

5. Notice what comes up and journal around it. Looking at the autobiography of our voice can help us to become more intimate with our voice and its lost notes.

Reconnecting with our wild voices

Talking therapy can be a wonderful space to explore the stories and feelings we have not given voice to. But, in my experience, there is only so far that we can get with rational speech. There are also wild sounds (and with them facial and bodily expressions) that want to cavort, growl and howl. Listen to a labouring woman's sounds, or someone in the throes of sexual pleasure, or someone keening for the loss of a loved one. These pre-verbal, primal sounds are part of our humanness, and yet there are few places in the Western world that they are welcomed. Breathwork and other sounding practices can help us to remember the wholeness of our voice, all its shades, textures, wild landscapes, vulnerabilities and power.

I remember my first retreat with Kim Rosen within the poetry and breathwork community I am part of, where sounding was a welcome, integral part of being in the space. This was when I got to feel just how inhibited my voice really was. Women would be sounding in the room and I was silent. My wild voice was buried under layers of conditioning. I didn't have the first idea of how to find it, all I could feel was the overwhelming stuckness that impeded my voice. Then, at the end of the week, I had my first breathwork session. This is a form of breathwork that uses a free form of breath, through an open mouth. The beauty of the open mouth is that any sound might fall out. Stopping the breath is one way that we hold back from our full expression. But when we breathe fully, the river of our energy system begins to unclog and all sorts of sounds can be freed. I had got through most of the session breathing but no sound had come. Then

Kim said in my ear, "sound" and this howl spontaneously came out. Effortlessly.

There are all sorts of wild creatures and sounds within us we have not met.

A few months later, I attended a La Loba retreat integrating Authentic Movement with Linda Hartley. I had not done Authentic Movement practice before and didn't know that they are traditionally quiet spaces. But now this wolf howl was freed, in a wolf woman weekend, the howl kept wanting to sound. Again, it was involuntary, but because others in the room were mostly quiet, each day it left me with very uncomfortable feelings of not belonging or being disruptive. Having spent so long not in contact with my voice, I could not and would not silence it, and in full respect of Linda as facilitator, she never once told me to be quiet. On the last day, we went into a movement session, and again, my wolf howl wanted to come, only this time, other women started to howl. As their howls sounded, my entire body relaxed. I lay down on the floor and rested, bathed in the sounds of their howling. It was a magical moment. The wolf, so long vilified, like the wild feminine, is actually a beautiful creature and for the wolf in me to feel her aloneness and then solidarity, was profoundly healing.

As women coming home to our instinctual selves, it is not unusual to find ourselves speaking the uncomfortable things, the things that are not being said, or making the sounds that are not being sounded. This is sometimes really hard.

Our wild voices want to be heard and loved, not
only by ourselves, but by the pack.

Over the years, I have reclaimed many of the lost notes of my voice and continue to do so. I also facilitate others finding their lost voices. This process that Kim Rosen calls the *"undressing the voice"* has been life-changing for me and many people I have worked with. I love this metaphor of undressing the voice, that chimes so beautifully with Inanna's stripping as she enters the underworld. What stiff suits and coats has your voice been dressed in? What heavy cloak wants to be taken off? What nakedness is longing to be revealed through the layers of your voice? And then how do we walk that wild voice back into the ascent, to speak with bold innocence what needs to be said?

The voice you once thought lost
will return to you.
Do not be surprised when you realize
that her tone is deeper, richer, and a bit
wilder
than the voice you remembered.
She has travelled
through the belly of the underworld
and while you spent your nights
plotting escape from captivity
she seasoned
in the dark recesses of the earth.

"The voice you thought you lost" by Sarah La Rosa

Gate Four – The Heart

When she entered the fourth gate, the gate of the heart, Inanna's breastplate was taken from her.

When the armour that covers her chest is removed, it reveals her most precious and vital organ: her heart. At this gate, she faces the loss of something that is so much a part of her sense of self, that she cannot imagine existing without it. The removal of the breastplate leaves Inanna's heart naked and vulnerable.

The psychological and energetic breastplate we each wear to protect our emotional selves is sometimes necessary as we grow and strive to live the life we think we are meant to live. Later, some of these ideals and ideas must be stripped from us, to bring us closer to our essential self. At the heart's gate we enter an existential crisis more humbling than we can comprehend.

What does life mean when we lose something that we feel is innate to our aliveness, to who we are? If we lose our country, a child, or our hopes of having a child, a loved one, a reputation, a purpose, or the life we imagined for ourselves...

The labour of the heart

For business coach, writer and podcast host, Sophie Jane Hardy, the catalyst was her journey through infertility.

> "I knew I wanted to be a mother all my life, it was never a question. And then, month by month, when I didn't become pregnant, that togetherness with life dissolved more and more. Until I began to feel I didn't trust life. Everything stopped making sense. It was a great maturation for me and it's an open wound that hasn't closed with having a baby."

To Sophie, being a mother felt like an inherent part of her life and when she had to face that that might not be possible for her, she felt that life had somehow abandoned her. Whatever the particular shape our unfulfilled dreams and expectations might take in a lifetime, these moments of loss are awakeners. They awaken us to longing, the most compelling and inexhaustible wanting that we ever experience. As I write this, I think of all those people who have gone on hunger strike, committed crimes of passion, or martyred themselves for something they love. What we love can bring us to the edge of death. People will bargain with their lives in pursuit of what they long for and believe in.

> *You can die for it – an idea, or the world. People*
> *have done so, brilliantly, letting their small bodies be bound*
> *to the stake, creating an unforgettable fury of light.*
>
> **from "Sunrise" by Mary Oliver**

The thing is, we can't bargain with the Goddess, with nature. As the Gatekeeper repeatedly tells Inanna, *"The ways of the underworld are perfect, they may not be questioned"*. The taking of the breastplate, then, is the obliteration of our most treasured beliefs about who we are, what we love and the way things should be. The removal of this armour exposes us to the unchangeable reality of our situation. It feels unbearable. But nonetheless, Inanna's breastplate is taken – there is no choice. Heart awakening always includes heartbreak and grief. But for me, even the term heartbreak is inadequate, though it is certainly a part of it. I say this because I have experienced heartbreak that did not strip my heart naked like the descent did. Heartbreak is cleaner, whereas whatever we are losing in the heroine's journey feels like a fundamental piece of ourselves being wrenched away. In that undefended space we keen, howl, pace, revolt, rage, surrender, fall, and then, in desperation do it all again. It is like a labour of the heart, one that won't let you stay still, but also one that renders you helpless to resolve it. As Sophie continues,

> "People would just say to me, 'Oh just let it go'. 'Just let it go' are words that should never be uttered to a woman who wants to conceive a child. There wasn't any letting go, it just didn't exist. It really wasn't an option. So, I get why Inanna has to go to the underworld, or I get whatever it was that pulled her down. There was a momentum that was happening, whether I liked it or not... I thought about it every day. It wasn't something I could pick up and put down. It was all-consuming."

This phrase *just let it go* or *you should be over it by now* are phrases that are often spoken with good intent, but show a complete lack of empathy. At some point, we may be forced to let go, which is the death part of the descent, but at this stage we are still compelled to hold on, to struggle, to pursue our heart's longing and when we are not getting what we desperately hope for, we suffer. Being all-consumed is a part of the energy of the heroine's journey. As Dawn Oakley-Smith, a facilitator of Equine Facilitated Human Development, elucidates,

> "Astrologically, it's very plutonic, it's Pluto, it's irresistible. It's the same energy that brings labour, it's the same energy that takes you to the toilet. You can't say to that – stop. It's a wave."

What both Sophie and Dawn's words point to is the unstoppable force that accompanies the descent. But this energy has a bit of the trickster about it, in that if the catalyst for the descent is the pursuit of something we long for, we may believe that because the energy is so compelling, eventually we will get what we want.

In chemistry, a catalyst is a substance that sets off a reaction, but the catalyst itself is not consumed in that reaction. This is highly relevant to the descent in that the catalyst is not always meant to be consumed, or had by us. This flies in face of the modern expectation that we should be able to 'have it all' if we just try hard enough or believe in it enough. In the heroine's journey, we often do not get the thing that we long for, at least not in the shape we hoped. We might be fooled into thinking, *if I want it this much, it must be meant to be.* But the heroine's journey is the pathway to maturity. In order to mature, we must come to terms with the fact not everything works out how we think we want. This is not always a story with a happy ending.

Even when someone has died, which is absolute and final, there can be some part of us at this stage that believes that if we hang onto grief itself, we will keep them close to us. So we keep saying yes to the pain, we keep risking our lives in the underworld, for the outcome we so hope for. Sometimes, as in Sophie's case, who eventually had her baby, it does take us there. But many times, the wave of the descent does not bring in on the tide that which we had hoped for.

The wild energy of the descent will not be dictated or tamed by us.

This is an initiation, and the thing common to all initiations is that they teach us that we are not in control: we will fall on bended knee, or flat on the ground, as many times as is needed.

The breastplate has, to an extent, protected us from life. When it is taken, we cascade down into the intensity of our feelings, desires and griefs. Loss of one thing unearths the torrent of all our feelings. It may begin with the catalyst, but once the heart is naked, we touch past griefs: pre-verbal grief (under two years old), ancestral, collective and archetypal griefs. We start with the personal and move way beyond into the bleeding heart of all things.

The river of our heart's losses is the river we must cross. It is vast, it is beyond what we can comprehend. At this point we necessarily cannot see how we will ever traverse it. You can't fight a river with a breastplate, it would just weigh you down. The breastplate's removal is our only chance of being carried by the river – it is the only way that we might find some buoyancy.

Suffering brings the rain of tears, because the rain of tears water the earth, because moisture on the dry earth of our being is guaranteed to bring forth new life. Tears are a river that take you somewhere [...] somewhere better, somewhere good.

Clarissa Pinkola Estés, *Untie the Strong Woman*

The death of who we thought we were

Though Sophie did eventually become pregnant, she was profoundly changed by her heroine's journey. She spoke to me about the stripping of her identity,

> "I was Communications Director of Tree Sisters and I was totally given to that mission for four years. But inside, I was stressed. It was stressful to be pioneering something like that, and to be so passionate about it. My system was getting too amped up. I could feel it. As a part of the descent, I had to face and heal a lot of chronic health challenges that seemed to be perpetuated by the stress. But it didn't seem to be enough. And I began to wonder if that role might have something to do with me not being able to conceive.
>
> I had to give up anything that I thought could get in the way of becoming pregnant. Which was a real wrench, because when Inanna takes off her breastplate and her crown, she takes off the things that show the world who she is, and the things that show her who she is. My work at Tree Sisters was a huge part of who I was, and I had to let it go."

One of the reasons the Dark Goddess has been exiled by humans is because, not only is she the bringer of life, she is also the bringer of death: the two inextricably linked. Rebirth cannot happen without loss, which is difficult for the heart to bear. Ereshkigal had already been calling to Sophie through chronic fatigue, which is the way many people get called to the descent. More recently, long Covid has rendered people energyless, unable to work and questioning who they are and how they live. Sophie could feel her system was too *amped up*. An amped up nervous system is so common in the spirit of our times, and is a feature in all the stories shared so far. We don't rest adequately, we are on phones till late, most of us are intravenously attached to our emails: it is normal to overwork and we are largely overstimulated. The oestrogen and cyclical nature of women's bodies makes us highly receptive to our environment. This can make us more sensitive to the override that is collectively happening in the modern world. Arguably, many of the illnesses we experience are a healthy reaction to living in an unhealthy world.

To enter the dark of the underworld is to enter the dark of the body and begin to hear what is going on under the noise. This calls us to make changes that are out of the ordinary for us, which those around us do not recognise as being something we would normally do. Inanna's breastplate is another symbol of her identity, royalty and worth in the upperworld: like the crown, the breastplate has an aspect of our belonging attached to it. As Sophie's names, when Inanna's upperworld objects are taken, she loses the things that show her and the world who she is. If we can endure the process, we can discover who we are beyond those identities. That does not mean that we no longer hurt. I actually don't buy into the old adage, 'everything happens for a reason'. Try telling that to a refugee who has been forced to leave their war-torn home, or a parent whose daughter has been murdered. Some things don't make sense, some things are incomprehensible and extraordinarily painful. But I do believe that something can come from the hurts we experience, something that is valuable.

As Sophie goes on to highlight, giving up her work with Tree Sisters did not mean she could stop working completely. She kept working, whilst navigating the descent. This is so often the case: we have to keep caring for those who depend on us, making enough money to keep a roof over our heads and all the while we are experiencing the biggest challenges of our lives.

> "I had to keep putting bread on the table and that's the dance that so many women go through that are in the descent. It's not like life will stop and wait. I see so many women are having to manage their careers around these things, and the world doesn't talk about it. Particularly with infertility. There is a biological reality for women who want to conceive, a time limit on when conception can happen and there are several things that amp up in the late thirties in potential health issues in the mum or the babies that are conceived. There is a ticking clock. But I feel like I am betraying the sisterhood by saying that. Because there is a feminist context, where we have been wanting to let biology fade into the background and create a system of equality. But I think we are now shifting to a place of recognising that there are differences (in men and women) that need to be recognised."

I feel this last point is crucial. In acknowledging her biological reality, Sophie felt on some level that she was *betraying the sisterhood*. This is a prime example of how, when the outer structures and stories do not support our inner reality, we have to adapt. And when we can't adapt, it can make us feel like *we* are the ones at fault. The removal of the breastplate is about meeting with the unchangeable realities underneath human ideals and constructs. There are many ways that women's bodies and women's experiences are different than men's. One of the fallouts of striving for 'equality' is that it has led to the myth that women should and can be the same as men, and do the same as men. A myth leads us to believe, consciously or subconsciously, that maleness is the one size that is supposed to fit all.

Many of us have unknowingly shaped ourselves to maleness for years. I certainly did. I thought I was clued up to it all, but there was so much that I did not see, which I even considered empowerment. As a young woman in my early twenties, living in London, emerging into the adult world for the first time, I now realise that I was trying to emulate the stories that the upperworld was selling me about being a woman. The ladette culture of the nineties was very focused on women being more and more like men as a form of empowerment, and I unknowingly bought it. I saw my period as a pain. I didn't want to be stopped by it. For so many years, like so many young women, I overrode my menstrual cycle, thinking the Pill was the best thing for me. I can now see that so many of the ways I was making choices were not from the inside, but were geared towards shaping myself to the outside world. My breastplate was part of the armour that made it possible for me to do this.

Over time, the girl-child becomes disconnected from the 'home' within her. Caught in the swirls of others, twisted in the shapes of others, depleted by the demands of others, she becomes outer-directed and loses touch with herself. Her breath becomes shallow. She ignores her body. She looks to saviours outside of herself for salvation and validation, forgetting the rich resources within her.

Patricia Lynn Riley, *Be Full of Yourself*

They say that home is where the heart is, the breastplate being taken then, is an essential part of the journey home. As we lose more and more of the armour that has enabled us to *twist ourselves* into the shape the upperworld demands, there is less and less to hang onto. We fall inwards, back into ourselves and the Earth. But 'coming home' to a body that is ageing, not doing what we expected it to do, or what we think it *should* do is very painful. At first, it doesn't feel like coming home, it feels like being wrecked. The heart is the gateway to failure, smashed perfection, loss and disappointment, all of which are doorways back into the home within us. As we come back into the body, we begin to recognise all the ways that we have abandoned ourselves, *we* abandoned Ereshkigal and let her become Queen of the Underworld.

Moving beyond self-abandonment

When I met my husband and we made our daughters, my heart opened in a whole new way. When I gave birth, I unknowingly rebirthed a part of me. One of the first things I said after my daughter swam out of my vagina and into the bath was, "Women are amazing!" Birth was a rite of passage that revealed a reverence and love for my mother, women and the feminine, in a way I had never felt before.

As the girls grew, I wanted to be an advocate for them. To become that, I had to discover how to be a better advocate for myself. I would have to learn how not to abandon myself. I define self-abandonment as all the ways that we exile our true feelings subconsciously or consciously (and usually a bit of both) in order to try to prioritise something on the outside of us, above what is really needed/ wanted inside of us. Usually this is driven by a core fear of rejection, ridicule, shame, abandonment...different people resonate with different fears. In trying to avoid the discomfort of saying what we really feel or need, we actually abandon ourselves. This is a form of defence supported by the breastplate. In reality, we don't avoid pain, the irony is that we are still in pain, it's just self-inflicted. Sometimes accommodation of others over ourselves is necessary to survive. But when unhealthy patterns of accommodation become habitual, meaning they play out without us even realising, we can get stuck in patterns of self-abandonment.

This keeps Ereshkigal in exile.

If what happened in the past is driving our responses now, this can sometimes debilitate, rather than help us. Our defences – our breastplates – are to be honoured and thanked. But the gate of the heart asks us to courageously feel what is going on under those defences – not to change the other, but to change our relationship to ourselves, so that we can welcome all of our feelings and bring Ereshkigal out of exile.

Uncovering the strength of the naked heart

There is something steely, structured, tidy and reassuring about the breastplate. Whereas, the naked heart is an entirely different beast. It is raw, sometimes irrational, often feral, and behaves in unexpected and unexplainable ways. A lot of what we feel at this gate is beyond clear definition, and a lot of what we lose in the descent might never be fully explained. We are commonly left with unresolved feelings that characterise the divine mess of the heart's gate. As Sophie illuminates,

> "Ours was unexplained infertility. We went through many tests, but there was no reason. And I wanted someone to explain why, so another part of my descent was, 'You can't have this, but I won't tell you why'."

Unresolved longing and grief can lead us to feelings of wanting to die, to losing faith in life altogether. As Sophie shared,

> "After three years, my sense of belonging to life really did start to crumble. I was depressed. I just couldn't understand how to be alive, if this wasn't going to happen. My relationship was suffering, the fights went on and on and on. I was having grief at every bleed, on the bathroom floor crying and my partner didn't know what to do with me. And then I would pick myself up again and do the next month and do the baby-making sex. Which is the least sexy thing in the world. Having to have timed sex, especially after three years – it really desecrated our sex life. Me as a fecund, sexual creature, that was something that dissolved. We forgot how to have sex for pleasure. It became functional and a failure."

In the pit of the descent something in us dies, and with it our *eros* energy goes to ground. Grief is exhausting, it takes so much energy that there is not a lot left for sex, or at least this was my experience. Also I noticed that when I did have sex, it brought all my grief to the surface which was difficult to feel. In the underworld, we enter the most lifeless place we can go without actually dying and we realise in a real, felt-sense that we are not immune to death and that not everything can be fixed. As Sophie highlights,

"I had to let go of the story that 'if you just try hard enough you can heal anything'. Or that plants can heal anything. Or alternative medicine or acupuncture can heal if we give it enough time and space. I had to let go of that, because it wasn't working and I was trying everything. I think I had a sense that there is an intelligence that orchestrates everything...and I don't know where I am at with that now. I think I am still in quite a dissolved state. But I didn't want to believe it. If that which orchestrates, was orchestrating this, then I didn't want it. It absolutely shook me to the core, it shook everything. I think there's a concept that if we're spiritual enough that we can make anything happen. A lot of prayers say, 'please make this thing happen for me'. But I now know that a real prayer is something like, 'make me strong enough to be with whatever happens'. Spiritually arrogant beliefs say that if you're pure enough, if you do all this deep inner work and heal yourself, that you will get what you want. This was my version of the Sky Gods, this was what had to dissolve.

It happens everywhere, and people think they're being kind, you know, when they would say, 'you know you will get pregnant eventually'. But I didn't know that. It's the vibration teachings, the Abraham Hicks, the teaching that we consciously create our reality. So the idea that if I could just think properly, I could create fertility...life is so much more intricate than that! The fabric of reality is impossibly huge to comprehend, how could it be as simplistic as that? I can't do with it, it's not big enough.

Another thing that had to go was control, because I was desperately trying to get control of the situation, but there wasn't any, and that was excruciating. Some women have to go through rounds and rounds of IVF and still don't get pregnant. There is no sense in it. We have this desire to package things into neat insights, but things don't make sense in this world. Which I guess is the laws of the underworld, that can't be questioned."

There is a New Age way of thinking that says we manifest our reality – I don't think we are that powerful. And furthermore, I think these are ideas rooted in white privilege. In their book, *On Connection,* poet and author Kae Tempest highlights,

> Behind every exchange and encounter, every missed chance or lucky break, behind every event or non-event in a person's life, there are entire weather systems, pushing for or pushing against.

The old myths are the antidote to the New Age, ego-centric ideals of contemporary culture. Initiations teach us that we are not in control and that we will be humbled. This is the process of surrendering to our humanness, not by getting it right, but by the virtue of getting it wrong. Self-care is so often sold as the nice things – the bubble baths, the spa days – but this is not the root of self-care. True self-compassion only arises when we feel our heart break for itself. This is how we bring Ereshkigal out of exile, by really feeling for her plight and recognising it as our plight. By being broken by our own impotence and mortality. The heroine's journey always means losing things that we dearly love – internally and externally – things that we think we cannot live without.

We all want to avoid pain, to make it disappear. What defines Inanna is her unswerving choice to go towards pain. Some burgeoning wisdom inside her recognises that she can't make Ereshkigal (her pain) disappear through exile. So rather than fighting, or running away, she goes towards the pain and allows it to soften, strip and season her. The breastplate may have given us superficial protection until now, but this gate dictates that we must learn from our wounds and to do that we first have to feel them.

The Divine Mother is often described as having a bleeding heart. Through Clarissa Pinkola Estés book, *Untie the Strong Woman,* I learned the story of Mater Dolorosa – the Mother of Sorrows – whose heart is pierced by seven swords: the hilts of which are said to be like the curling sepals that protect the buds of the heart. The story tells us that with prayer and time these rose buds will burst into flower, again and again. The loss of the breastplate opens us to the wounds of the heart so we can release the tears that water these flowers. Without the armour of the breastplate, we move beyond romanticism, beyond idolatry, through and beyond our personal pain even, until all that is left is the vast, resilient, indestructability of Love.

Eventually, Sophie went for IVF treatment, which was successful first time round. She expressed great gratitude for that, but also spoke to the unhealed wounds that she is still carrying.

> "The IVF worked first time and now I have Arty. So I would have
> imagined that I wouldn't feel grief now. But I just started my period
> five days ago for the first time, and it was a huge wave of grief. So it's
> not gone.
> There's a Greek myth of Chiron – the bull that has a spear in his
> side – and the spear has to stay, the blood has to keep flowing for the
> wisdom to flow. So it's this idea of the wounded healer, that we have
> to be wounded to bring any healing into the world. My experience
> means we can have this conversation and hopefully I can meet others
> who are in grief who might feel a sense of belonging with me."

Sophie was the second woman who mentioned the wounded healer in my interviews. This story has a resonance with the seven swords through the heart. Inanna must meet her wounded self in order to mature, but also so she can be of service. Wounding allows us to form the connective tissue of grief that connects us to all things. Our hearts' losses are an essential part of this path.

> *Grief offers a wild alchemy that transmutes suffering into fertile ground. We*
> *are made tangible and real by the experience of sorrow…In a very real way*
> *grief ripens us, pulls up from the depths of our souls what is most authentic in*
> *our beings. In truth, without some familiarity with sorrow, we do not mature*
> *as men and women. It is the broken heart, that is also capable of genuine love.*
>
> **Francis Weller, *The Wild Edge of Sorrow***

I feel this wild alchemy that Weller describes comes through the heart of our longing, and without death we cannot reach it. The longing that poets write about is the driver for change, creativity and connection. It is so difficult to articulate the pain we feel in the heart. At this time, for me, poetry was one of the only things that could express what was otherwise indescribable. As Stanley Kunitz names in the poem "The Layers",

"How shall the heart be reconciled to its feast of losses?"

Pinkola Estés tells us that the swords through our hearts are *not* the ones that caused our wounds, but rather they are the swords of strength that we earn through our struggles. This is oppositional to the breastplate, that seeks to protect the heart from wounding. This gate teaches us that the heart must be wounded to reveal our sacred strength, to uncover the hidden meanings and learnings of the descent, to help us heal, to carry us towards new life, to lead us to our courage and open us to Love. To walk through the gate of the heart is a calling to live with integrity and maturity and face the most difficult aspects of being human. Grief slows us down and rearranges our perception of everything and in doing so clears a pathway between the spirit of the times and the spirit of the depths. The crack in our hearts is the place where the microcosm of our personal losses meet with the griefs of the wider world. When the two interweave they might guide us towards action.

Devotion and the call of the heart

Walking the path of Love, is like walking over a chasm of fire on a bridge of hair.

An early Christian mystic via Irina Tweedy, *Daughter of Fire*

This is the path we walk when we live a life of devotion. I believe the heroine's journey is a path of devotion. But not devotion to only light and perfection, but to the totality of our experience, dark and difficulty included. Inanna has to come off her upperworld throne, be stripped naked and then impaled on a meat hook before she can rise rooted in the Earth. This idea is mirrored in the Christian tradition also, whose central symbol is a naked, bleeding man whose arms are pinned open, his heart ruthlessly exposed.

What Gate Four leads us to is relationship with the source inside of the things we lose. Our heart is stripped of its armour so that we can land in the arms of our true nature, the thing underneath our lives that abides. The thing that is untouched and indestructible, that poet Juan Ramon Jimenez says, *"will remain standing after I die"*.

The cross is an energetic embodied symbol of the heroine's journey. As humans we reach out through the heart, but to support this we must also to reach down into the Earth and up to the sky. In my own life, it was so natural and easy for me to reach out through my heart. But I was not rooted energetically into the Earth enough to support the energy of my heart. This led to unclear boundaries and a tendency to give too much of myself away, too easily. Many women and girls are not rooted in their sex, the wisdom of their cyclicity and the Earth and as a result our hearts are not properly supported. If we cannot root into ourselves, we can end up on an inexhaustible search for rootedness outside of ourselves, in all the wrong places.

The animal quality of the heart chakra is said to be like a black musk deer that exhausts itself running after the smell of musk that it loves, never realising that it is the scent of its own belly. Capitalism exploits the nature of the heart and sells us the idea that what we love and need will be found in the perpetual outwards search to quench the thirst of our desire. Whatever form that shows up for us – a drug, money, fame, followers, a person, a role – like the musk deer, it exhausts our heart as we grasp for things on the outside. The secrets of our longing are actually held in the musk of our own belly. This is especially poignant for women, whose cyclical wisdom held in our wombs, has been so shamed. At some point, like the exhausted musk deer, we have to stop racing around trying to do, be and have it all, and see what happens when we stop and meet what is inside of ourselves.

In Stephen Cope's book *The Great Work of Your Life* he looks at the necessity of the life/death/life cycle. The whole book is devoted to exploring the notion of dharma or a calling in life,

> *Our understanding of dharma today is obscured by our fondness for the cult of personality and for self and celebrity. Our understanding is obscured by the narcissism of our time [...] The primary distortion in my dharma life has been the age old misery of self-absorption. Deep in midlife I had begun to feel the awful burden of wanting to be special; wanting to be better; wanting to experience every possible adventure in life.*

As Cope names, we *want everything,* and Ereshkigal is there to teach us that that is not possible. This yearning to be special and have everything can actually block the flow of life. To let go of the upperworld *cult of the individual* and admit that we are just like everyone else: this is a key teaching found in the losses of our heart. We are unique, yes, but we are also ordinary. So, Ereshkigal takes our breastplate and with it, the part of us that wants to transcend the ordinary in an attempt to supersede our own impermanence. In this she is ruthless, whether we survive or not is inconsequential to her. In nature there is no separation between life and death, they are necessarily and unequivocally intertwined. Whether we die or live, we will be composted into the whole.

I realise now that, in many ways, Ereshkigal's indifference is the greatest love we can be offered. In my experience, loving presence is a willingness to be alongside another or ourselves, even in the face of death or suffering. Therefore, in the absence of the Ereshkigal's preference, something within us is allowed to go.

Even in her darker aspects, in what scholars call the chthonic, or earthy, she is still portrayed as part of the natural order. Just as all life is born from her, it also returns to her at death to be once again reborn.

Dr Rianne Eisler, *The Chalice and the Blade*

This path asks us to face ourselves again and again, layer by layer, so that we can breed compassion to the deepest depths of our being. The root of the word compassion is *compati*, from the Latin that means 'to suffer with'. It is rarely easy.

Listening to the heart

Take a moment to put your hands on your heart and check in with how your heart is feeling in this moment.

If your heart had a voice, what might it say?

How do you honour your heart? How do you not honour your heart?

What is your experience of devotion? What are you devoted to?

Take a moment to attune to the heart and see what arises from your heart's own wisdom.

Gate Five – The Solar Plexus

Suddenly it was clear to me —
I was something I hadn't been before.
It was as if the animal part of my being
Had reached some kind of maturity that gave it
Authority, and had begun to use it.

from "Saint Animal" by Chase Twitchell

My true power should come like a shoot
A force of nature, no pushing, no holding back.

from "Dedication" by Rainer Maria Rilke

When she entered the fifth gate, the gold bracelets were removed from Inanna's wrists.

As we move below the heart's gate, we enter the subconscious landscape of the solar plexus, symbolised by Inanna's gold bracelets. Gold because this is a fire centre in the body, but also because gold signifies Inanna's upperworld wealth and power. At this gate we ask, what does it mean when we lose our power, social standing, status and visibility?

What does it mean to feel invisible or powerless?

This gate calls us into a new relationship with power. Somatically, the solar plexus is the place from which we navigate and assert our personal power. In the dominator dynamics of the upperworld we are encouraged to seek power over. Power over nature and the Earth, power over other people, power over our bodies, and so on.

Many of the well-known hero mythologies support this paradigm and end in the hero killing or overcoming some representation of the wild feminine and suppressing the emotion and heart of the masculine. This is the kind of power we have been taught to aspire to. Medusa has her head chopped off, Sedna has her fingers chopped off and is left to drown, the Selkie's sealskin is stolen and the dragon is always slain. The underlying message given to us in these mythologies is that the dark, wild, chthonic feminine, like Ereshkigal, must be killed, exiled or vanquished in order to come into our full power. But, if we always employ our inner masculine to oppress our wild feminine we enter an internal war within ourselves. This war can perhaps be won, we can dominate aspects of ourselves, but at a cost. This myth calls us into a remembering of what it means to have 'power with', because power is always relational.

In the dominant paradigm in Western culture, where power is aligned with domination systems, it is assumed that one must choose between strength and compassion. Indeed, choosing one or the other is simpler. However, the greatest ally to using power with skill and wisdom is the ability to bring power as strength together with power as compassion.

Cedar Bairstow, *Living in the Power Zone*

I believe the Inanna-Ereshkigal myth is one of the oldest known stories of 'power with'. Not because it excludes violence or conflict, in fact because it includes the darker energies of our humanity and offers us a teaching on how to integrate them as a part of our humanness. It shows us that empathy, compassion and creativity can forge a pathway into relationship with the darker parts of ourselves and our humanity, so that we can broaden our capacity to be all that we are.

Power rooted in strength *and* compassion is perhaps more complex, but that doesn't mean it is not possible. There are other myths that also teach this for example the Hindu myth of Kali and Shiva (see Chapter Eleven). Paradoxically, it is only when the heroine is humbled and stripped of the objects that are associated with power in the upperworld, that she can feel her relationship with power from a new vantage point – both her own power and the power of others.

At this gate we uncover all the ways we have been powerless, as well as awakening to the ways we are powerful. When her gold bangles are taken, Inanna begins to question what strong actually means. Vulnerability as strength is a core teaching of the descent – an idea so contrary to upperworld heroic ideals.

The excerpts at the beginning of this chapter are from poems that were companions for me as I reckoned with my own power in the underworld. In my heroine's journey, *the animal part of my being* that Chase Twitchell refers to was first initiated through giving birth to my daughters, but then I had to descend much further to learn how to walk with that authority into the rest of my life.

My devotion to becoming an advocate for my daughters unearthed a devotion to the service of the feminine and women. As I entered my authority as a mother, I was asked to wake up to all the ways I was dancing to other people's tunes. This process not only served my children, but my own evolution and my work.

At this gate, in my work and my parenting, I faced
square on the fear of all the things I felt I didn't know
how to do, or that I felt I wasn't allowed to do.

I now realise that this not-knowing was essential: it signified my arrival in virgin territory, yet to be revealed. On this path, what we are meant to do and be is revealed to us, not the other way around. This is the feminine rite of passage, but I feel it is amplified for women living in patriarchy, because, we have not got the entire writings of history to support our evolution now. On top of that, when we start working to our natural rhythms and a more feminine way of being we step firmly out of the mainstream. The heroine is one who is initiated back into relationship with the wild feminine. As we explored in Gates One and Two, not knowing is an essential part of the rewilding process. The creative right side of our brain flows, it does not pin things down. It is about being and moving. It is only by moving we can remember and relearn its ways. The scripts we have introjected from society and those around us might say, *you are going mad, you are an imposter, you are a terrible mother/space holder/manager/wife/person…*

The fire of this gate purifies our perceptions of self.

When we step into our power, many relationships will likely be challenged. The fire of the solar plexus lights up anywhere where we have been overly compromising and have not yet individuated. Individuation is the process of beginning to know ourselves as separate from the other, be that another person, religion, culture, community, work, family narrative… The process of individuation calls us to be more and more true to our own inner compass. To be Inanna in the first place, we are probably already pretty firmly stood in our own shoes. But the exiled parts of us, those parts which have not yet been parented to full maturity, the Ereshkigal parts, are likely still playing out survival patterns from childhood – these parts must now also individuate.

As I entered the underworld, the relationship I had with key authority figures in my life started to shift in profound and challenging ways. As my gold bracelets were taken, so too was my high-achieving, good daughter, rigid, perfectionist self. The residual scripts from the past that were confining me began to burn off. Because these scripts often come from our nearest and dearest, our closest relationships are rattled by the furnace's flames. A huge fear when this happens is that we will be left alone and that we will not survive. But if we are going to step fully into that animal authority, we have to take the risk and let the shoots of our power sprout up out of the ground, to see what we truly look like.

The removal of the gold bracelets is a catalyst for unveiling the shadows and power dynamics at play in our relationships.

In our family systems and relationships, power dynamics are so familiar we often don't notice them. The root of the word 'familiar' is from the Latin for family. What is *familiar* or *familied* in us, is so much a part of us that we don't know any different. The fire of Gate Five sheds light on all of this and initiates us to find out who we are underneath these relationships, underneath the roles that have shaped us, and that we have shaped ourselves to. Whatever is burned off is fuel for the fire and whatever stays is transformed in the process. As Carl Jung said,

> *The self is relatedness [...] The self only exists in as much as you appear. Not that you are, but that you do the self. The self appears in your deeds and deeds always mean relationship.*

As we start to consciously feel our self in relationship to those around us, we get to notice, in real time, the places we shrink back from speaking out, the places we feel rejected, right through to the places we are welcomed and supported, and the feelings that come up for us in relationship to all of this. There are many places that we compromise in order to keep relationships on an even keel, and sometimes this is necessary. But sometimes, the compromise is too much. This gate might require us to risk some of the relationships that mean the most to us.

An exercise for thinking about how we adapt in our relationships

1. *Think about the relationships in your life. Which relationships are most supportive? Which relationships challenge you the most?*

2. *Then, returning to the exercise on the voice from Gate Three, take a poem and read it out loud. See what you feel and notice.*

3. *Then, think about someone in your life and imagine them in the room as you speak the poem again. Notice: does your voice change? What does your body feel like? How does your breath move? What do you hold back? What is invited out more? Anything else you noticed?*

4. *You could repeat the process a few times, imagining different people and see how different people affect you. If you want to take it one step further, you could ask to try it out in real time with someone that you know and see how your voice and body feel in the presence of different people.*

It feels important here to underline what I named at the beginning of the gates: the descent does not happen sequentially. My descent was actually a continuous succession of relational shifts with different people in my life and at the centre of that was my changing relationship with myself and Source. It's not as though you enter this gate and all your relationship changes happen and then you move on. The changes taking place in our relationships reverberate through all of the seven gates, and our rising, forcing us to ask questions about how we navigate our personal power within our relationships.

The split self

In a world that has very clear pathways to power, a world that rewards and prioritises the voices and bodies of some more than others, this gate also brings many collective and structural issues to the fore. We do not start on a level playing field. As women, how do we navigate personal power in a world that is not structured to include and respect us? I spoke to author and founder of Womancraft Publishing, Lucy H. Pearce. Lucy is a neurodivergent woman, living in a neurotypical world. I spoke to her about her descent,

"I am a late diagnosed autistic woman. I was late to be diagnosed because I am very good at masking. I am very good at being friendly and charming outside and you know, not being too weird... And very much scripting and doing huge amounts of research before I do anything so that I feel safe. But when I put my work out there, I'm putting my raw, autistic, true self out, without the masks. Which is terrifying. Especially in a local area where I work so hard to mask myself.

There is this deep vulnerability that I will be seen and judged. I have experienced this so many times through my life, without realising why it was happening or what I was doing wrong. I didn't know I was being (in other people's eyes) strange, I didn't know I was autistic, I was just being me. I didn't realise that these were parts of myself that I had to censor and hide. So the self that I could show in the world got smaller and smaller over my lifetime.

My books are like the flipside of that, which is liberating and freeing for myself and so many women who read them. And at the same time it's an absolute psychological battle, because I am going against every one of my safety mechanisms that I've built up over the years. It's more than the normal inner critic that most people have to deal with, it's battling with the psychological safety mechanism of being neurodivergent in a mainstream world. And that really takes its toll."

When the stories in the outer world do not reflect our internal story, we can end up feeling like Lucy, that we must hide ourselves. But what I feel Lucy describes so clearly is how the authenticity of her creative process renders her naked, like Inanna, and the deep vulnerability of that. Whatever these heroine's journeys are, they are not a fairy story: our most painful experiences are caught up in these journeys. When I reflected this to Lucy she replied,

"I think our culture focuses on the glorious starts and the wonderful finishes, when you get to be queen. But you don't see the walking through the forest of thorns having your skin ripped off in between. You can see even in the media and public response to tennis player Naomi Osaka: we want to praise the person who has overcome mental illness, but we don't want to see someone struggling in the middle of it. We don't want to see someone's vulnerability and weakness. But most of our lives is the mess, is in the thorns, is the tricky navigating of that dark path through the woods, down underground, with no one really to witness it, no one to share it with. This is so much of the baseline of my writing. I want to hand on both my lived insight and the information I have churned up in the process because, fuck it's hard, and no one is talking about it."

The upperworld doesn't like to acknowledge our human mess. I think so much of women's lives and experiences have been sent to the underworld for fear of shaming, or ostracisation. Women have been split in two: what is allowed to be seen and what must not be acknowledged. This split manifests in all the gates on some level.

Supporting the solar plexus – Rising rooted

In the last chapter, I spoke about the need for rooting down so we can open our heart to embrace life. Being rooted is also important for the solar plexus. Somatically, if we cannot be rooted in the depths of our experience, through our pelvic bowl, our legs and down into the Earth, then we may end up over-compensating by projecting out beyond our centre from the ribs (sticking our ribs out). This is a somatic expression of being over-identified with others. It is also a way of striving to be seen in the world. Literally our upper body goes forwards and up and we leave our lower half, our underworld – Ereshkigal – behind. If we try too hard to assert ourselves from the ribs, we create tension which disconnects us from the back body and the root chakras, which support the solar plexus as the effortless power centre of the body. This lifting from above the centre, rather than through the centre, can reflect patterns of *over giving* or *giving ourselves away*. It can also be an attempt to get what we want from the outside, rather than from a place of internal integrity, like the musk deer in Gate Four.

Conversely, if we are so beaten down that we cannot lift through the mulch of the underworld, we may get stuck down in it. We may lose contact with our personal power altogether, collapsing down into the ribs, thereby denying the fullness of our own aliveness, breath, body and expression. I feel this striving upwards, or collapsing downwards, can be exaggerated in women because of the lack of support in the world for power rooted in the deep feminine. If we are shamed from the roots of ourselves and our bodies, then we have to strive to find power from a higher centre which is much harder work. This pattern promotes a split between the upper body and lower body that disconnects us from our roots. Either way, if Inanna is not rooted in Ereshkigal, she has to work twice as hard.

Where can women find healthy models of empowerment in a world that has such a distorted relationship with feminine power?

Misshapen power

For women in the West, many of the symbols of power or source are usually personified by males, which can further disenfranchise us from our own power. As Mary Condren elucidates,

The absence of empowering female images (the dominant cultural symbol systems) both reflects and effects the subordination of women. The very lack deforms the way our drives are constructed so that both body and soul are put in the service of the patriarchal social order.

This gate initiates our return to the nature that we are, the Goddess within, our connection to source. The divine feminine is actually embodied everywhere we look. Once we recognise her, we begin to see her everywhere, hiding in plain sight. She becomes reflected in vulval shapes in the bark of trees, the unapologetic voluptuousness of flowers, the sensuousness of catkin buds, the ripe rolling breasts of hills and in the sensuality of our own bodies.

The Sky Gods live in opposition to this, within us and externally. We are encouraged to dominate and tidy our wild natural beingness. The nature inside us and outside of us is undervalued in the upperworld. And when we get the reflection that we are not valued by the Sky Gods, it influences how we shape ourselves to get the power we need to survive.

This shaping, misshapes women.

Facing our fear of the Sky Gods

As Inanna enters the fifth gate, she reckons with her true power and distortions of power on the inner and outer. I spoke to Lucy when her book *She of the Sea* was just being released,

> "*She of the Sea's* very heart is my final putting to bed of the Sky Gods and owning my relationship to the sacred feminine and magic. There, I said it: magic. The term 'Sky God' is one I use again and again in the book. In my world the Sky Gods were the patriarchal institutions. We have had a very challenging time over the last few years with one of our children who was undiagnosed autistic, who was beginning to struggle harder and harder. It's something that I picked up and went to the first Sky God who was the GP who said 'no, nothing to see here'. So I went back again, because they are the gatekeepers. And again I was met with disbelief. You have to have the right words to open the bureaucratic gates, and without those words from the Sky Gods, the lived experience of the person is deemed non-existent."

The medical profession and our academic institutions are places where the Sky Gods sit and decree who has power and who will be respected or helped. These institutions also teach us in all sorts of ways what is of value in the world. Whatever we turn to the authorities for, be that help with our health, a crime, money, we have to turn back in the direction of the strong Father (women can embody this as much as men) and hope that they will help. But, as in the myth, the Sky Gods are not primed to help the feminine, and so there may be many ways that we end up, like Ninshubur, knocking on the door of the wrong Gods for help. As Lucy continues,

"Until that point, I didn't know what autism was. I only knew what it was perceived to be in our culture, you know, non-verbal boys or 'Rainman'. I didn't know that it applied to one of my children, I didn't know that it applied to me, I didn't know that it applied to my mother. But I knew that there was something different about me. In my early mothering years, I had this constant awareness that there was something different or wrong about me and my ability to function. Something that I needed to hide from the Sky Gods, from the authorities, so that I didn't have my children taken away from me. And it wasn't because I was a bad mother; it was because I didn't function in the same way as others, and I feared that that could be read as being a bad mother. My family are everything to me, so when I found myself having to ask the Sky Gods for help it was very frightening. But they wouldn't help anyway, because they didn't believe me.

When you are in the most vulnerable place of your life and you find yourself having to ask the people that you're most scared of, that you have spent your whole life avoiding, to come and help, it is horrific. And then they said no. And then you have to turn yourself inside out to try and persuade them why their help is needed. I wouldn't wish anyone to be in that position. I now know that women around the world are in that situation with kids who are awaiting diagnosis for all sorts of things, who are awaiting judgement from on high and are going hearts in hands begging for help. Help from the people who are judging them. People who have the power to take children away. Who have the power to give or not give medication, to give or withhold support. And what makes it worse, is to know their help isn't even the best thing, but that it's the only thing available at that point, and then to still be turned down... Well, we did that dance for eight years, two and a half years intensely."

Many people face arduous processes to receive help. Without the money to pay for a private therapist or doctor we are in the hands of the Sky God public institutions and they have the power to do as they will. For people of colour there is an additional layer to this, in that unconscious bias is still incredibly prevalent in all our institutions. This has been highlighted by the Black Lives Matter movement and the brutal unjust murders of people of colour in America and other parts of the world at the hands of the Sky Gods. The people working in our institutions sadly do not always show up in the Enki or Ninshubur form that we desperately need. Eventually, with some family help, Lucy and her family found a private doctor who was their Enki.

"He was a kind human being, who also works within the public system. He saw us and he got it straight away. I trusted him. So after paying for my daughter's diagnosis, I approached him about a diagnosis for myself. He said he would help me in exchange for a painting, because he knew money was tight. For me, to exchange something from my creative soul and spirit, which is so impacted by, and yet empowered by, my neurodivergence, to make an exchange from that depth of myself, for the words (the diagnosis) that I needed, was very meaningful. He is a wonderful man, who is doing great work and is able to go between the worlds of patriarchal medicine and the people on the ground who are living this, with deep respect. And he does so without taking away any of your personhood. He is someone who has the capacity to acknowledge the real struggles that you have, whilst completely holding the respect for you as a person."

In the Inanna story, when Ninshubur appeals to Enki for help, he uses his creativity to conjure the *kugarra* and *galatur*, little creatures made from the dirt underneath his fingernails, who he sends to the underworld to empathise with Ereshkigal. Enki has dirty fingernails; he is not the pure, white, sitting on a cloud Sky God. He is a gardener with a playful twinkle in his eye. He is in contact with his dark feminine and, I believe, his own wounding which enables him to help others.

In my experience, facing the Sky Gods and our fears about them, whether those fears are real or imagined, is essential. Even being abandoned by the Sky Gods might be essential. In a sense they have to fail us, in order that we enter our relationship with power in a new way.

We have to lose God.

Discovering that we can survive without the Sky Gods' approval or presence, is eventually fortifying and liberating. By the time Inanna comes to Gate Five, over half of her upperworld garments have been removed. In stripping these aspects of herself, she is stripped of the upperworld ways of knowing her own power and gets to feel, as Lucy did, how she is subject to the power of others and how she navigates her sense of agency in the midst of that. It's a messy journey that takes us into the institutions within and without, to meet our power anew. It is not as simple as rejecting society entirely and going to live off-grid to assert your personal power (though it may look like that for some). For the vast majority of us, our initiations involve learning how to live in our integrity, authenticity and uniqueness *within* a world that encourages us to compromise and accommodate in ways that are not healthy for us. For Lucy that meant continuing to write and create despite her fears,

> "I recorded this journey as I lived it and it became my book, *Medicine Woman*. It was my way of staying sane as I was navigating it all. Writing was my way of integrating and giving voice to the silenced parts of myself and being witnessed in that. I included many women's stories, placing my own in the context of the collective women's experiences of Western medicine, so that they – and I – knew we weren't alone."

Our creative endeavours can empower us to resurrect Ereshkigal and offer a potent and tangible way of witnessing ourselves, and being witnessed by others.

Beholding and being beheld as a form of power with

We can enter the role of witnessing another like a Sky God, from above. Some 'expert' authority figures such as: medical consultants, religious leaders, some therapists, teachers, parents even, may take this stance of power over. Or we can stand beside others as a witness, in partnership. What is the difference? It can be very apparent or very subtle. As a therapist and space holder there are many ways I can take power or, make choices that are a conscious endeavour to share power. For example, it could be asking the client what they feel or notice, before I weigh in with my observations. It is trusting the other and entering an enquiry together about whatever is unfolding, as opposed to standing in a place of superior knowing before we even begin. This gate asks us to become more sensitive to the ways we relate to power internally and externally. Lucy reflected on being the witness and being witnessed,

"Being able to hold space for someone in the descent and being able to witness it and help be their strength when they need you to be, but without trying to take it away from them has been a learning curve for me. Because I have always been a fixer. I have always tried to take everybody else's struggles on myself. Or I have been scared by other people's struggles, and have tried to hide from them because they're so intense and I feel them so deeply. But being able to witness and hold space for someone you love as they are descending is, I guess, what you would call maturity. Not taking their suffering personally, but truly acknowledging the depth of it and loving them through it and trusting that process for them, is a state of maturity that I think you can only offer when you have done it yourself. It is what any good therapist does. It should be a ritual, an initiation: you have gone through that cycle, so now you can hold space for yourself and others to do the same.

Descending and rising should be celebrated, not in an ego polishing way, but because it's one of the biggest human accomplishments you can make, bigger than a doctorate or an Olympic medal."

The doctorate and the Olympic medal are, in a sense, the Sky Gods' ways of rewarding achievements they value. But we don't usually get a gold star or a title for the heroine's journey. In fact, we probably lose more titles than we gain. It often lands with us to name and value our heroine's journeys. It takes the greatest courage to step through this fifth gate and embody the fire of the solar plexus, to stand for the possibility of a different way.

To re-write the narratives about what being heroic actually entails.

We need more people to recognise these rites of passage as they occur, and behold others as they move through the gates of the underworld. To own our failures and struggles has not been the way of the upperworld, though this does seem to be changing. It is becoming more and more normal for well-known people such as Meghan Markle, sportswomen Emma Raducanu and Simone Biles to name their struggles. These role models owning their experience helps to normalise our heroine's journeys.

Social media has its downsides, but it provides a witnessing space for stories that would not or could not have been seen and heard before. Lucy continues,

"The witness is vital to me. For me, the primary medium is writing, in journals and books. But I have discovered that giving actual voice to my words is the final part of the work...When I listen to the audiobooks that I have recorded, I get to witness my work in a way that you don't when you're reading it with your eyes. I remember author Jennifer Louden saying, 'Make sure you always take your own medicine. What comes through you, is first and foremost for you.' I thought that was a really valuable point, because when you're doing this work often the focus is on the audience, but actually, no, you owe something to yourself to take the nourishment of that into you as well, once it's finished. To stand soul to soul with your work and not judge it in your head, but actually experience it. We are very well trained in how criticise our work and improve it and judge it. But how do you witness the essence of that work and allow it to touch you? How can you be changed by it, rather than you trying to change it? That is true witnessing."

In any public-facing creative work, we must enter the nakedness of being witnessed – both internally and externally – which is potent ground.

For me beholding and being beheld by another can be one of the purest examples of *power with* the other and both people might be changed by the experience. One of the things we do in the group work I hold is eye gaze. To gaze into the eyes of another human being, without words, only looking, is a profound experience. It is a highway to connection, beyond our masks, beyond our upperworld self. Gazing into the eyes of another can transport us into another realm of being in minutes, sometimes, seconds. So often we enter relationship with a sense of knowing. Eye gazing, for even a short time, can undo our grip on the known and land us in the realms of being with another.

Please note: Some neurodivergent people can find eye gazing particularly challenging and so the exercise given here may not suit everyone. But if you feel the willingness to try it, it can be a very rich experience.

Eye gazing with yourself

Find a mirror and sit with yourself. Set a timer for three minutes and gaze into your own face and eyes.

Look at your own face as if looking at a work of art. Notice the shape of your mouth, eyes, nose, skin... If judgement comes up include it and then drop in the question: what else is here?

Then focus specifically on your eyes. Notice all the different the colours in your own eyes. And then dive into the black hole in the centre of your eyes.

Notice how you are breathing? Holding the breath is one way we hold back feelings, see if you can allow a few breaths to move as you look.

Notice what you witness about yourself and what arrives in your awareness. Then take some time to journal about it.

Coming into a new relationship with power and boundaries

When Inanna individuates from whatever she has become entangled with, she can start to see herself and her relationships through new eyes.

A big part of my descent was learning about right relationship: with my family, my teachers, my work, my students, clients, the world and myself. Through it I learned how to be in relationship without being consumed and how to exist in my own power without unhealthy dependency on others. And conversely, I also learned how to be more vulnerable, and how to lean into support when I most need it. It isn't all about self-sufficiency, nor is it all about leaning off our own centre and becoming totally dependent on the other. It's about getting to know how to pendulate between these polarities. Coming into a greater sense of both our independence, and our need for support.

What we are talking about is boundaries, and these are a life-long learning. It can be so tempting to think of boundaries as fixed entities, I often hear people say *I know where my boundaries are now.* I feel it is a little more nuanced than that. As we discussed earlier, relationships are living entities and therefore, boundaries are alive within them. It is important that we don't fetishise our boundaries, but allow them space to breath and space to 'get it wrong'. Sometimes, as the saying goes, we have to be had, to know we've been had. This is one of the most useful things I know about boundaries. Often the way I get moved to a new edge with boundaries is when one is 'crossed'. And mostly I don't feel that until after the fact. But each time it happens, I get to know my edges a little more clearly.

Power, nuance and the mystery

In Western culture the Sky Gods still hold most clout. They are the forms of authority that are valued and recognised: the bankers, lawyers, consultants and the media. In the pandemic, this hierarchy was momentarily challenged: carers became the heroines. It would have been so good if there had been more economic reward for the nurses, doctors, midwives, care home assistants, cleaners, teachers, shop workers, all those who kept the world going through Covid. But sadly, the Sky Gods will not relinquish their power, or their gold, willingly.

The societal structures we live within contain huge power differentials, which impact our relationships with our own boundaries and power. These external factors have to be included in any discussion of power. The heroine's journey asks us to wake up to all the internal and external power differentials at play in our lives. Power differentials are inbuilt in the dominator model, creating a system that requires us to fight for our place. So collectively, if half of us are lifting up from the ribs and exiling Ereshkigal to get on top, and half have collapsed into the poverty trap – what is our collective energy doing? Burning out and over-working simultaneously. Those who get paid the most, are often the ones who have adapted best to a maladapted system.

We are a sick society, we need to take the veils off and start to address the trauma patterns held within our collective structures.

In our world, power is mostly seen through what we have, rather than what we surrender. But it is only through Inanna's willingness to surrender her upperworld status, that she can meet Ereshkigal. Then, both receive the gifts of the relationship, both sisters grow. Sometimes, difficulty can strengthen and deepen relationships. As humans we have a huge capacity to draw together in the face of adversity. In the descent, we come face-to-face with our own humility and vulnerability, which allows us to develop more compassion and this changes our relationship to power. Without an empathic witness, without acts of kindness, in times of challenge we tend to default to the certainty of the strong Father again. Even if we are disempowered, at least under the dominator we know where we stand. Ironically, the poorest and most vulnerable people have a tendency to vote for their own oppressor. At this time of populism and polarity it can be easy to lose sight of the other's point of view. But as we compost our crown, we enter the myriad of possibilities at play in any given scenario and as we enter Gate Five and the final gates, it is imperative that we learn to hold nuance.

My anchor is love. It is life sustaining to understand that things are always more complex than they seem. This is what it means to see clearly. Such understanding is more useful and more difficult than the idea that there is a right and wrong, or a good or bad, and you only have to decide what side you're on. In real love, real union or communion, there are no simple rules.

bell hooks

The interplay of opposites often creates conflict in our relationships, in ourselves and in the world. But discord can help us uncover what is in shadow. To grapple with and face this calls us to mature. One who descends is looking for another way and we have to return to the wilderness of our own complexity to forage for it. This gate, like all the others, holds paradox. When we enter Gate Five, we are called to step into our personal power, whilst paradoxically recognising that we are but one small part of something so much bigger. Here we continue to widen our view to the horizon of the Self: that which is beyond family, beyond name, beyond status.

Jung believed that the Self is always present, and that the ego grows out of the

Self. In other words, we arise out of the mystery. He also believed that Self always retains its mystery, that it is never fully known. More recently, Ian McGilchrist in his book *The Matter with Things*, stated that the Self can only be known in motion, it is never fixed. In this way, the only way we can truly experience it is in real time, when we are *relating*. Relationship implies that something is fixed. But really, every interaction is new. It may have connotations of old patterns inside of it, but in reality we can only be in relationship in the moment we are relating to each other. As we enter the shadow realms of the underworld, that which shape shifts, changes and moves, within us and around us, teaches us. But not by us fixing it down, but by dancing with it, and surrendering to it dancing us.

Like Jung, I feel that we emerge from what is constant and indestructible. What becomes 'I' emerges from something much greater and more mysterious than 'I' can possibly comprehend. Therefore, what we call 'I' is part of the Mystery, Source, God or Goddess, Nature, whatever your particular name for it is. This is what we might catch a glimpse of when our gold bangles are taken from us. At this gate, we meet with the power that moves through us, that which is us, but is also greater than us. As Rilke so clearly tells us, "my true power should come like a shoot, a force of nature." The upperworld asks us to distort, push or hold back this power. But in the underworld, our true power is revealed to us. When there is nothing left to hold onto, that which endures and emerges is the source of our true power. At this gate, the ways that we have misshapen ourselves in relationship to power start to unravel and be revealed. We discover that the vastness from which we spring does not need us to misshape ourselves, that vastness is actually asking us to be fully alive.

Gate Six – The Womb

I talk to my inner lover and say why such rush?
We know that there is some sort of spirit that loves
the birds and the animals and the ants
perhaps the same one that gave radiance to you
in your mother's womb.
Is it logical you would be walking around entirely orphaned now?
The truth is you turned away yourself
and decided to go into the dark alone.
Now you are tangled up in others and have forgotten
what you once knew.
That is why everything you do has some weird failure in it.

Kabir translated by Robert Bly

When she entered the sixth gate, the measuring rod and line were removed from Inanna.

Chakra six is the gateway to our sexuality, creativity, womb, sacrum and our emotions. Associated with the water element, it is the place where we feel and flow, and can freeze and stagnate. As we have already been establishing, living in a patriarchal world is to live in a world dominated by a narrow set of masculine ideals, models, rhythms and measurements, meaning we can feel like we are failing as women when our cyclical nature asks us to move differently. As the Kabir poem finishes, *that is why everything you do, has some weird failure in it.* Girls and women are set up for 'failure' because we are living in socio-cultural structures that are not designed with us in mind. One place this is felt deeply is in our wombs.

The womb and pelvis are the heart of a woman's creativity, the muddy soil from which the shoots of our creativity springs. Even if a woman's womb has been removed, in Traditional Chinese Medicine it is thought that the energetic centre of the womb still resonates in the body. Having worked with women who have had hysterectomies I have found this to be true. The pelvis and womb are also the underworld of our bodies, where the energy of our hurts, traumas and unprocessed feelings reside.

The Inanna and Ereshkigal phases of the menstrual cycle

The womb is the sacred container of potential new life, and it is also the place from which we release what is ready to die. The life/death/life cycle of the heroine's journey is held in the microcosm of the menstrual cycle. In our fertile years, the majority of women move through the four seasons of menstruation monthly. Our moontime is winter, after which, post-bleed, we enter the renewal of spring. In the peak of ovulation we are in the summer of the cycle, and then as we enter autumn, we begin the descent back towards our bleed in winter when the unfertilised egg is released, along with anything we are letting go of from the previous moon cycle – this is the death part of the cycle. These are the four seasons of the menstrual cycle as taught to me by Jules Heavens who names,

> "Recognising the seasons within the menstrual cycle brings several potent threads to the surface. It allows women to find the gifts of difference in each phase, as well as supporting us in transitioning through our life and our life's seasons. It brings us back into connection with our wild and instinctual animal self and nature."

The founders of Red School, Alexandra Pope and Sjanie Wurlitzer Hugo, use this model with the addition of the *via positiva*, which is the upward energy of the first part of the cycle and the *via negativa*, which is the downward energy in the second half of the cycle. I like to think of the *via positiva* as the Inanna part of the cycle, and the *via negativa* as the Ereshkigal part of the cycle (see diagram).

The descent is a super-magnified version of this cycle, where we enter the *kur* and die to what we have outgrown. As Inanna enters the Sixth Gate she is like an almost leafless tree at the end of the autumn. What remains of how she measured herself and what she thought she knew, is now hanging only by a thread.

The Ascent and Descent of the Menstrual Cycle

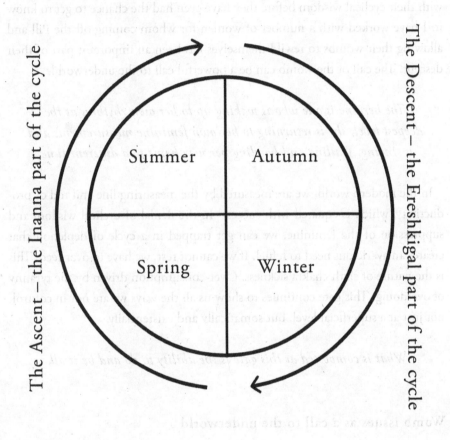

Our calendar is based on the Gregorian calendar, which follows the solar year. Whereas lunar calendars are based on the moon's cycles. Not all, but many women's menstrual cycles, also tend to follow a lunar cycle, hence the name: moontime. In this way, conscious menstruality is a reclamation of the feminine measurements of time. But this is still not the dominant teaching in our society. Menstrual shame is endemic and colours the way women feel about our bodies. So many women are put on the Pill during adolescence thereby losing contact with their cyclical wisdom before they have even had the chance to get to know it. I have worked with a number of women for whom coming off the Pill and allowing their wombs to rewild themselves has been an important part of their descent. The call of the womb can be a powerful call to the underworld.

The heroine is one who is waking up to her own rhythms at the deepest level, she is returning to her own feminine measurements and is singing, wailing and howling her way home to a different tune.

In the modern world, we are measured by the measuring line and rod of productivity, which is equated with success. In the denial of cyclical wisdom and suppression of the feminine, we can get trapped in a cycle of depletion that creates an avaricious need to refuel. If we cannot rest, we have to over-feed. This is the nature of sixth chakra sickness. Over-consumption driven by the tyranny of overdoing. This gate continues to show us all the ways we are not in control, not just at a superficial level, but somatically and existentially.

What is composted at this gate is the ability to do and be it all.

Womb issues as a call to the underworld

If we negate our feminine rhythms, we become entangled, as the Kabir poem so beautifully illustrates. This might show up in dis-ease in the body, burn out, stress, menstrual cycle pain or chronic fatigue. For psychosexual somatic therapist, Kalia Wright, it showed up as a loss of vitality, which eventually led her to discover that she had endometriosis, a condition where cells similar to those of the womb lining start to grow outside the womb.

"I had an awareness that something wasn't quite right with me for a number of years. I experienced a loss of vitality, which was really upsetting and unnerving. At times I would despair, because I didn't have the answer, I didn't know what was going on. There are a lot of unknowns in the journey with endometriosis because it takes up to seven years on average for people to be diagnosed with it and a lot of us don't present with painful symptoms in that area. For a long time, I had this deep sadness because I would look in the mirror and see a lack of life. I couldn't see the life moving in me and that echoed into my confidence, my expression, it really impacted how I showed up. That brightness, that spark, just got smaller and smaller and smaller till I couldn't see it anymore. It was a huge process of grief around losing the brightness…and all the while, I just saw my hair getting thinner and thinner, I could feel my bones getting achier and my skin was getting duller and duller. I felt like a death was occurring in me, physically, there was a real receding of life occurring in my being at the time."

Kalia's loss of vitality was taking her into the descent to reconnect with her womb, to reconnect with Ereshkigal. Like Inanna, she made the choice to follow the moan and made changes in her life.

"I changed my life, I quit my job, I thought maybe stress was causing it. I started to radically shift how my outside world was looking to make space for a bit more flow, a bit more ease. That was a courageous decision. It took all my might to give up everything I have known for fifteen years to really honour what my body was telling me, which was – 'something's not right'. I didn't know what just yet, but I knew I needed to make space to listen. In the masculine energy of patriarchal society, I couldn't listen closely enough because I was too busy. I had got hooked into the cycle of, 'I have got to do this job for money' and I didn't know anything different. But I had to say enough is enough."

As we have seen in the other stories in the book, overwork is a recurrent theme. If the masculine inside is not holding a supportive structure for our inner feminine, he can become our internal slave driver, the one who keeps us going no matter what. As Kalia names,

> "I learned a lot from endometriosis. For me, it landed first in my relationship to the masculine. I was a highly yang person, lots of outward energy: do, do, do; plan, plan, plan; got to get this done; no rest. There was no time for the softer, more feminine or yin parts of me, no time to rest. I was relentless and that's how I was socialised to be: 'you've got to achieve', 'you've got to do', 'you've got to progress', because that's what it means to be successful as a woman. I had chronic burn out, caused by the lack of contact I had with good boundaries, the lack of contact with my needs. All these things over the years had brought me into this process, and endometriosis taught me that I had to get into right relationship with my boundaries and my needs."

When we cannot voice what needs to be honoured on the outside, the other alternative is to oppress it on the inside. In the groups I hold, one of the invitations is to dance with your womb and let her lead the dance. Some women find they have a really strong reaction to this, some women say things like, *"I don't want to have a relationship with my womb, it's given me nothing but pain"*. I don't want to idealise menstruation, like many things in life, sometimes our bleed is painful and inconvenient. But I believe this is exacerbated by living in a culture of menstrual shame and suppression. It is painful to have a womb in a world that does not support wombly rhythms. So, Ereshkigal, embodied in our womb, becomes our scapegoat, the one we reject and blame. What some women meet when the masculine measuring rod is removed is the war we have been having with our own anatomy and needs – the tyranny of our own internalised oppressor.

The menstrual shame that seems such a part of Western society is a matter of culture at war with nature. For members of other traditions, we hear again and again about the value of feminine bleeding and menstrual seclusion.

Barbara Tedlock, *The Woman in the Shaman's Body*

With an MRI scan they found a two centimetre cyst on Kalia's left ovary and possible signs of endometriosis. In the six months that followed Kalia's symptoms worsened significantly,

"It seemed like my body felt like, 'now it's okay to start expressing signs of endometriosis'. My body started to speak and it got really, really loud. I then started to go into shock that I might have endometriosis and that it might not be curable. I was feeling a lot about not being able to control this and coming to terms with the fact that this might be my future. I was reading a lot of stuff on the internet that was quite negative and I felt, I don't want this for myself. So I was chronically stressed and there were other things going in my life that were adding to this really intense incubator of…trauma, I would say it was traumatic. My nervous system was fried and I just felt really burnt out which was exacerbated by lockdown."

Ereshkigal's moan got so loud that Kalia contacted the doctor again and asked for another scan. They discovered that the cyst had grown from two to thirteen centimetres and decided to operate.

"It all came to a head when I got the surgery date. That was where I got to the death process. The point where I completely surrendered to the fact that my life might be completely different when I came out of that surgery. Because they couldn't see what was going on in there completely, and because the cyst was so large, I had to sign a consent form basically saying that they would have to go with what they found. And that consent form was not pleasant, I wouldn't have wanted any of that for myself.
So, on the day of the surgery, I went into this process of speaking to my body and doing some consent work with my body. So I was sat there and saying, you know, 'There are going to be surgeons around here in these parts,' (signalling pelvis and womb area) 'and potentially entering my vagina to put in various things and we have got to know that it's going to be difficult, but I am available for this. We need to do this, because it's going to help going forwards and we need a break.' My body was just screaming at me, 'we need a break, we need

a break from all this.' So my body was really onboard with it. I knew there was the potential that I was going to lose an ovary, that I was going to be infertile, potential that my bowel or bladder might be impacted… And I don't know how many people are connected to themselves the way that I am, to feel all of that.

I would just sit in front of my surgeon crying and asking lots of questions. And I said to him, 'This is how I am keeping myself resourced to have this surgery, so you don't need to do anything about the fact I am bawling my eyes out. You just have to give me space, so that I can function. I need to let this move, because if I go into this surgery holding it all, that's not going to be good for my prognosis coming out. I need to shift this through.' So it was good that I also felt empowered to express myself. And then the final bit, was on the hospital trolley going into the theatre and praying. I think it was the biggest test of trust in my life."

The kind of trust Kalia is referring to is the unconditional kind. It's easier to give trust with a condition, with the underlying message of *"I trust you to do what I want"*. What the heroine has to mature into is unconditional trust, which accepts that whatever comes, she will meet it. As Kalia elucidates,

"Surrender was a big deal for me, because I have been super-independent and able to control, but I couldn't do that in this situation. It was a complete surrender and actually more of a submission: I learned the art of submission in this process. Surrender was more of an opening and a kind of receiving and an accepting of what was going on. But submission was a reverence and a willingness to bow down to the lesson the universe was teaching me. There was an awakening of something else that was different."

The phrase *bow down* is exactly how Inanna appears to Ereshkigal – *bowed low*. Submission humbles us to the powerful forces at work in our lives, that we cannot control. As the Gatekeeper says, *"The ways of the underworld are perfect, they may not be questioned"*. Kalia continues,

"Endometriosis was the accountability partner that I really needed. Me and endometriosis are in relationship now, because I respect my endometriosis as a teacher, because that's where my body will tell me when I am out. I had to really get clear and change how I was doing things. Learn to be more vulnerable in my day-to-day life. And, you know, it's a great quality of mine, to be super-confident, super-dominant, super-assertive, really powerful…but, there's also a part of me that needs to be soft and tender, to receive and be more in my vulnerability and openness. That was the lesson that endometriosis taught me.

The crux of being able to soften was about me not rejecting the masculine anymore. So I discovered it was both: I am very masculine, and I was also rejecting the masculine as well. I used to be very anti-patriarchy but because I was using the same masculine energy to fight patriarchy, I was adding to the same energy, which actually wasn't helping…When I softened, I was able to notice that underneath, there was this deep hatred and mistrust of men. I thought I didn't hate men, because I felt we were all impacted by patriarchy, you know, men too and non-binary people. But I have since realised there was another part of me that was rageful and hated men. And I thought, 'Wow, I need to sit in that.' And when I did, I realised that I was holding such contempt, and whilst that was in my body, that level of subconscious resentment that was in my underworld, whilst I couldn't see that, it was creating this effect in my body. I think it was a physical manifestation of bitterness and resentment."

Here Kalia describes her meeting with Ereshkigal, who holds our unmet rage and hate. Once she could turn towards it she discovered,

"I realised that under my hatred was a deep fear. You know, logistically as a woman, I can't fight a man off and that was a big fear that I didn't want to touch into. So my go-to was to project that outwards and hate men and keep them at a distance. But what that meant was, I wasn't really having any meaningful connections with men in my life, I wasn't really loving men, or ever trusting men. For me, healing happens in connection, and I thought, if I am not connecting with men, then how am I part of the solution? I can be angry at patriarchy but what am I doing to change that? But I didn't want to shut down my contempt and my anger either, because that's valid as well."

The rage that Ereshkigal is holding is both sacred rage and it has a shadow (see more in Chapter Nine) which I hear Kalia name so clearly here. It is humbling to contact the level of contempt and hate we feel and the way this might have been acting out in our lives. On the flipside, rage is a vital aspect of our *eros* and to shame it, is to suppress an essential aspect of our life force. At this gate we must admit the darker emotions, from our vulnerability all the way through to our own cruelty and rage.

One of the things I was so moved by in Kalia's story was the way that her relationship with her surgeon called her into a new relationship with a male figure – an Enki figure. Having not trusted men, to be put in a place where her womb and reproductive health were in the hands of a male consultant seems to me like an important part of Kalia's initiation.

"He was really empathetic with my situation and his commitment and care was great – he was solid. It would have been easier for him to lop off my ovary. But I said 'No, I want to have babies. You can't do that. I am not willing to give up my ovary'. I told him, 'I would like you to do your best to save my ovary, and if you really can't then I trust that that's the decision you're making'. So it was me seeing that he was a collaborator in my journey, not the power in my journey. I was empowering myself, through seeing this as a co-creative relationship, rather than a patriarchal doctor that I just have to do what they say. I don't do that anymore, they are guides on the way, but I am not giving them my power.

I saw the other consultant in the hospital and he just wasn't the same, so I feel very blessed to have had my surgeon, someone who listened. You have all manner of feelings when you have had such an intense surgery – I was under for over five hours, it wasn't small – but the care that he took to show me the photos after, he just took such care and you could feel it."

Kalia found her voice, and in doing so, it seems that she actually called this consultant into his creativity, into the Enki aspect of himself. Just as, in a sense, Inanna's courage to descend calls Enki into his creativity. Here we see another example of how being listened to, cared for, heard and respected by a male authority figure can be profoundly important on our heroine's journey. In this journey, we have to allow all the feelings we have towards males and patriarchal abuse, and from here, we can start to form a new relationship with the masculine on the inner and the outer (see more on this in Chapters Eleven and Thirteen).

Contacting the mother wound

Collectively, the overriding of natural laws and the subordination of the feminine has created a split in the psychospiritual and somatic life of not only women, but all of us. We are nature and nature is us. To deny this is to orphan ourselves from Mother Earth. And for women to deny our wombs, is to deny the Earth inside of us. Entering Gate Six is an Earth initiation. When we really allow ourselves to enter the personal grief of what we have done to ourselves and what has been done to us, we also open the door to the wider grief for the Earth. As the poem at the beginning of this chapter asks, *is it logical you would be walking round entirely orphaned now?* The truth is, we haven't been orphaned, yet. But if we continue as we are, then, like Dumuzi, we may well have to be sacrificed.

What we meet as we enter the underworld is not only our father wound but our mother wound: the ways we have rejected and split off from our own mother, the Earth and/or our inner feminine. One common reaction to patriarchy is to reject the mother in favour of the father – preferring to become our 'father's daughter' and reject the traits of our mother. Or our mother may reject us, feeling fears of being usurped by her daughter's youth and womanhood. In myths we see this personified by the stepmother in Cinderella and the Evil Queen in Snow White, both of whom try to thwart their daughters coming into the full majesty of their womanhood. Even in the Inanna-Ereshkigal myth, it is not female elders that Ninshubur appeals to for help, it is the Sky Gods, the masculine, who she turns towards.

The heroine's journey may include a healing journey with our actual parents, but this is not always possible. For many this means we have to grieve what our parents did not have the capacity to meet within us. We must let die the striving for our relationship with our parents to be different than what it is/or was (if our parents are deceased or estranged from us). In the process of acceptance, we can become our own internal parent. I don't know if we ever fully heal the mother or father wound inside ourselves. But we can grow the capacity to behold the parts of us that needed their attention and begin to measure ourselves by our own ways and means, rather than our parents'/societal/partner's or anyone else's expectations. As the myth teaches us, the agency to heal the split lives inside of us.

Reconnecting with what we truly desire

Everything we do not want to feel, or cannot bear to feel, we put down into the underworld of our pelvis, with Ereshkigal, and there it stays. The problem is, our pleasure and life-fullness also lives in our pelvis. This chakra is the seat of our desire and *eros*. Culturally, we have a very difficult relationship with desire. The norms and values of Western culture shape how desire is measured. Some desires are deemed as being more socially acceptable than others. Like in Kalia's story, the desire to *do, do, do* is praised, but the desire to rest is not. These narratives influence what desires are allowed and what we suppress. At this gate, the lapis measuring rod is symbolic of how we measure what is of worth in society and which desires are valid. Some addictions are praised, such as helping, whilst others such as drug addiction, are not. However they manifest, the roots of our addictions come from the underworld of our wounded self. These coping strategies may have helped us survive for a while. But Inanna has started to outgrow them, which is part of what subconsciously compels her to descend.

> *Ereshkigal's moan calls us back to the root cause of the*
> *pain so we can begin to reclaim our desire.*

The split between Inanna and Ereshkigal can perhaps be most clearly seen in the split of female sexuality. On the one hand, women are expected to be desirable and sexually alluring, whilst on the other hand, we are not supposed to be 'too brazen' and must certainly not be 'a slut'. The patriarchal view of female sexuality is problematic. In the Bible, Eve was held responsible for Original Sin.

With the rise of Christianity, any woman in her power or sexual sovereignty was viewed as a source of evil.

All witchcraft comes from carnal lust, which in women is insatiable.

**Malleus Maleficarium (*The Hammer of Witches,* the
Catholic Church's official witch hunting manual)**

Even in current times, the impact of this runs deep. In a sense, Eve is the mother of all women, rejected because she was responsible for the fall of humanity. Her sexuality was a sin and a problem. I believe that this narrative is intrinsically woven into the embodied psyches of all of us. Like so much of women's experience, the story of our anatomy and pleasure got lost and distorted through his-story. We in the West are caught between feast and famine in our sexual discourse. On the one hand, we are hypersexualised as a culture: pornography and advertising exploit feminine sexuality. We are saturated with ideas of what sex should look like, feel like, sound like and how to 'perform well'. All of this can disenfranchise us from our own unique sexual expression and contributes to a culture of anxiety that masks and stifles the true embodiment of our sexual expression. At the other extreme we have the culture of silence, 'don't talk about it', 'don't be too sexual', 'don't have sex before marriage', 'don't have sex this way, only that way'.

*To reconnect with our authentic sexuality can be
an underworld journey all of its own.*

There is now a shift towards women reclaiming our sexuality and pleasure. And I feel there is a move, certainly in younger generations, of exploring beyond the traditional confinement of patriarchal, heteronormative paradigms of sexuality. But pornography, much of which exploits women and creates an online space for the abuse of women to be normalised and fetishised, poses new problems for all women. We are still taught to look to the male gaze (whichever sex is perpetuating it) for approval, acceptance and validation of our sexuality, attractiveness and expression. And the media tries to keep women who step outside the box in their places through public shaming and vilification.

*Many of us internalise this male gaze, seeing ourselves from the
outside in, rather than feeling ourselves from the inside out.*

For many people that I work with, moving away from a performance-centred version of their sexuality and beginning to feel their sexual energy from the inside is an essential part of their heroine's journey. To remember how to be guided by our own pleasure and body is one way home.

Dancing with your womb and vulva

Follow this link to the Descent & Rising playlist on Spotify: **tinyurl. com/wombdancing** or create your own.

To begin place your hands on your womb. Take a few deep breaths into your hands and pelvis. Imagine you are filling your pelvic bowl with breath. Breathing into your vulva, labia, clitoris, cervix, womb (or where your womb was), ovaries (or where your ovaries were). Then, when you feel ready, begin to move from this place. Follow the dance, let any sounds and emotions out that want to come. When you finish, take some time to rest.

Then, when you feel ready, pick up your pen and journal about how that was for you.

What did you feel?

What was difficult?

What was pleasurable?

Anything else you wish to name?

You can repeat this practice on a regular basis as a way of listening to your vulva and womb.

Inanna is a Goddess of sexuality: she has agency over her own body. She *chooses* to go to the underworld because something inside her own intuitive wisdom senses that it is necessary for her journey to maturity. In the Persephone myth, which is a later patriarchal adaptation of the Inanna myth, Persephone is taken to the underworld against her will and is raped by Hades. She is initiated into her sexuality by him. However, it hasn't always been like this, as Clarissa Pinkola Estés elaborates,

> In these old religions the maiden need not be seized and dragged into the underworld by some dark God. The maiden knows she must go, knows it is part of divine rite. [...] In the time of the great matriarchies, it was understood that a woman would naturally be led to the underworld, guided there and therein by the powers of the deep feminine. It was considered part of her instruction, and an achievement of highest order for her to gain this knowledge through first-hand experience.

Inanna models a different possibility for women as sexual creatures in our own right. Even before her descent, Inanna is a sexually empowered woman. There is a whole verse earlier in the poem as translated by Diane Wolkstein and Samuel Kramer, which celebrates the sexual union of Inanna and her husband, Dumuzi. The verse shows Inanna as a woman who knows her own body and pleasure. She sings to him,

> "My vulva, the horn,
> The Boat of Heaven,
> Is full of eagerness like the young moon...
> man of my heart, plow my vulva."

The sensuous directness of Inanna is so contrary to the virginal feminine of the Christian faith, as it was adapted by patriarchy. Where, as we touched on earlier, the feminine is split into the chaste Virgin Mary and the whore, Mary Magdelene. The wholeness of a woman and woman's sexuality is lost in this ideology, whose stories have shaped so much of our cultural and moral measurements. We have been held in a split that keeps Ereshkigal in exile and Inanna elevated in the sky of perfection. To allow the wholeness of our sexuality to be rediscovered and remembered, is a doorway to higher knowledge rooted in the fecundity of our own root. This is what Inanna symbolised, pre-Eve, pre-patriarchy, pre-dominator society and we can follow in her footsteps to find our way home.

The *eros* wound

An essential part of my heroine's journey was healing the split from my sexual self. It was a coming home to eroticism as a way of living and recognising that *eros* is the creative energy that fuels everything, not just sex but my work, cooking, raising my daughters, writing – it's my life energy. Anodea Judith explores,

Eros is an ancient god, the connecting force that unites and delights, bridges and soothes. In Hindu mythology, Eros is the god Kama, the originator of all the gods, the binding power of allurement that holds the universe together. Since the force of Eros brings things together its denial can pull things apart. In culture this leads to destructive activities. To embrace eros is to have the capacity for surrender, to be able to flow with the biological nature of the instinctual/emotional body.

This flow is literally embodied in the fluids of the body and pelvis, be that the flow of sexual fluids, the blood of menstruation, the flow of urine as we empty our bladder, the flow of amniotic fluid when we birth, and the flow of our tears. The sixth chakra is associated with the water element. The sea has a depth and wisdom and is often associated with the feminine. The flow of our emotional, sexual and moon cycles are inherently linked. What we deny becomes stuck or frozen. When we remember to listen to the flow, the ice caps of the freeze begin to thaw.

I believe part of the freeze originates from the trauma of living in a misogynistic society that has abused and controlled our feminine nature and bodies for so long. Entering Gate Six is a reckoning with this, that awakens us to all the ways that it is true in our lives. The female body and female sexual pleasure is often commandeered by men, for men. Meaning that many women subconsciously internalise the notion that our bodies are for others, rather than for ourselves – this impacts our entire relationship with *eros*. When we wake up to the painful fact that we have been colonised, we often experience, grief, shame, anger and a whole host of emotions.

The erotic is a resource that lies deep within each one of us…It is deeply rooted in all of our unexpressed and unrecognised feelings…when I speak of the erotic then, I speak of it as an assertion of the life force of all women. Of that creative energy empowered, the knowledge and use of which we are now reclaiming in our language, history, our dancing, our loving, our work, our lives.

Audre Lorde, *Uses of the Erotic: the Erotic as Power*

As Anodea Judith outlines above, denial of *eros* can pull things apart, but paradoxically it also pulls us towards whatever we have not admitted. It attracts us towards the wound so we can tend to it: this is the path of the heroine. What I have discovered in myself and in beholding many women as they journey back towards sexual wholeness is that it isn't the light-filled, orgasmic journey we initially hope for. Before we ascend, we have to descend. Entering this gate requires that we compost the measuring stick the Father gave us and replace it with our own unique tempos and designs.

There are many ways that societal narratives and ideals can lead us to measure our sexuality against the prescriptions of others, rather than feeling and embodying our sexuality from the inside. Releasing ourselves from this confinement may help us to uncover whole new realms of our sexuality. Which could include: opening to new sexual experiences and sensations, owning your sexual identity, sloughing off shame about your fantasies, discovering for the first time that you even have fantasies, saying what you don't like, indulging in self-pleasure and so much more. Whatever way this configures in your life, coming home to your own beauty, abundance, turn ons and utterly unique sexual expression can be a vital part of the heroine's journey: a reclaiming of our own erotic being.

> *Follow no authority –*
> *but your own true nature*
> *Make a sacred fire*
> *and throw on it all that you would use to harm yourself*
> *Make kindling from shame*
> *Let your dance be wild*
> *Your voice honest*
> *And your heart untamed*
> *Be cyclical*
> *Don't make sense*
> *Initiate yourself*
> *Initiate yourself*

from "Dear Woman" by Aisha Wolfe

The heroine's journey an erotic initiation, that happens at its own tempo, in slow time, in the spirit of the depths, in the earth of the body. It measures us, not the other way around. And when our roots are strong enough, our *eros* will rise.

Gate Seven – The Root

When she entered the seventh gate, her robes were removed leaving Inanna completely naked.

The base chakra is about our relationship with our bodies and our lineage: both our ancestral lineages and the lineages we create as a continuation of that. Therefore, any unprocessed ancestral trauma is held in the root. It also includes any spiritual lineages we may be part of. And it is about the land we are native to, the place we live and the animals and people that we commune with there. In short, it is about belonging: to ourselves, to others, to the mystery and the Earth.

On an embodied level, many of us, if not all of us, have a core wounding of this chakra and it can start as early as birth. If our mother's body felt unsafe due to circumstance, abuse or ill health, then this wounding can happen before we are born.

At this gate we reckon with our core root
wounding and make it our teacher.

As Inanna's robes are taken, so too is the last vestige of identity and connection with her upperworld self as she has known it to now. When we disrobe we become nameless from all the names we have held. Who are we when we lose our belonging to whatever we thought we belonged to? It is simultaneously a maturation and a return to innocence like no other. There is a beauty in this and it is almost unbearable, because nothing can be the same again.

When our robes are taken, we become naked to ourselves. What renders us naked, in large part, is not only what has been physically lost through the seven gates, but also the disarmament of the old defence mechanisms that we previously relied on to cope with those losses. The removal of the robes is the ultimate humbling. Whatever strategies we have used to patch up and cover the parts of ourselves that we didn't want others to see and that we couldn't bear to see, are gone. Though uncomfortable, this is essential if we are to truly reveal what we have previously been unable to admit. In the acute defencelessness of our nakedness we enter new relationship with our bodies, our environment and our roots. It's a seismic shift.

What and who can we trust when we are totally naked?

She who must not be named

My vagina is a shell, a round pink tender shell, opening and closing, closing and opening. My vagina is a flower, an eccentric tulip, the center acute and deep, the scent delicate, the petals gentle but sturdy.

V, *The Vagina Monologues*

The female body is still taboo – especially the vulva. For women living in a patriarchal world, our 'down there', as two female doctors only very recently referred to my vulva, is still a problem. It largely exists in exile, unnamed, in the underworld, like Ereshkigal. And yet, it is exploited everywhere, in a culture that feasts on the female body and yet disrespects it at every turn. Therefore, to descend back into the body is a subversive act.

> *The world tells us to reach higher to do more*
> *and to achieve impossible ends. But we know we must plummet deeper if we*
> *are to become*
> *– rather than seek –*
> *The Holy Grail.*

from "The Roots of a Woman" by Edveejee Fairchild

The descent is a process of feeling the incarnation of our wounding. We can tell our stories again and again from our minds and yet still stay on some level disconnected from the body. To finally be able to *feel* the energy of what is somatically held within us, gives us a real relationship with Ereshkigal, in the here and now. The magic of this is, that we don't necessarily even have to know, or look directly at what happened in the past. We simply have to remember how to listen to the felt sense that is here right now and the rest will unfold. Through Maureen Murdock, I learned that in the oldest original Grail legend, Parsifal, who is on the quest for the Grail, doesn't attain it by force, battle or domination. He attains the Grail by asking the compassionate question, "What ails thee?". This is what we must ask our body as we enter Gate Seven. All the gates teach us how to unconditionally listen to the body. Because the body remembers.

We know beyond what we know.

This is also the way we remember how to follow our implicit memory, that which is written into our subconscious somatic experience, so that we can uncover the wisdom of our trauma. It is an act of subversive surrender to tend to the body in this way. It is the practice of listening, feeling and importantly, allowing, that is synonymous with the feminine. At Gate Seven we are asked to enter into conscious partnership with our bodies at the deepest level.

Vagina is the word most commonly and wrongly used for the entirety of our female sexual anatomy, which in itself is problematic. The vagina is only the canal up into or out of the female body. The etymology of the word vagina is "sword sheath" meaning that in the English language, the root of the word for our internal anatomy, is in itself defined by an external source – the penis or "sword" that it is presumed will enter it. The naming of women's bodies has come through male-centred discourse. Not totally surprising then, that female sexual pleasure and energetic anatomy is still woefully misunderstood, not only by men, but by women too. Our vulva, labia, clitoris, womb, ovaries, vagina, and cervix are all significant areas of a woman's sexual anatomy that come together to form the root of the female body, and orchestrate the full array of our sexual pleasure. When I first started holding women's circles, every time I said "vagina" I got red hot, there was so much energy in my body around saying that word out loud. Why? Because there is ownership in naming our body and there is a power in our root.

For generations now women have grown up with the abused, shamed and degraded "vagina" as a normal aspect of our culture. The Inanna myth was written in a time before this was the case. As named in the previous chapter, Inanna openly and freely delights and revels in her own sexuality, body, vulva and her sensate aliveness: in this, she has medicine for us.

Though sexuality is generally associated with the sixth chakra, in reality the last two gates are very difficult to cleanly separate. Uma Dinsmore-Tuli offers insight into an additional chakra at the base of the female body called *yonisthana*.

Yonisthana cakra[*], literally means the 'special land of the womb' or 'the place of the cosmic gateway'. Yonisthana is an additional feminine refinement in our understanding of the cakra system, the womb's special place where water and earth meet in creative fusion.*

---

[*] Uma Dinsmore-Tuli uses the sanskrit spelling of chakra.

This intermedial chakra recognises something important about female embodied experience. It describes the fertile synergy of water and earth at the base of a woman's body, that gives us the capacity to be simultaneously rooted and flowing. Our vulvas can also be messy and Gate Seven is a holy mess. If illness or birthing a child is our gateway to this chakra, it may ask us to get up close and personal with the messy nature of our bodies, which inevitably at some point in life, will refuse to behave as we want and expect. I feel *yonisthana* also highlights the energetic and physical impact of having a doorway into and out of our bodies, which means that woman's outer environment is so deeply felt in her inner world. Unlike males, we are not sealed to the outer world in the same way. We can be penetrated deeply by our environment, our experiences, our own fingers and our relationships, which affects our psyche, nervous system and somatic experience. When we acknowledge this and feel it, we can become both sturdier and more tactile to our own permeability as women. At first this may feel very vulnerable. But as we have seen at every gate, the strength of the feminine is her vulnerability. Knowing this as a physical reality is one way we can grow deeper connection to our roots.

The roots of female divinity and spirituality

Inanna is a holy priestess of the temples, therefore to disrobe her is to remove her spiritual authority. The fear of being disrobed, whatever this means to us personally, is one of the things that keeps us in check. Patriarchal religions encourage us to renounce the body, especially the female body which is seen as 'the root of all sin'. Even in yoga lineages, the female body has largely been ignored in favour of practices and language that prioritise the male body and energetic experience. This is changing now, as many women are starting remember more cyclical, female honouring ways of practicing yoga.

Historically, the female body has been treated as male property. This has been encouraged by the Church through Bible stories still told to this day. For many years, I felt alienated from religion because of the misogynistic nature of it. But my angry rejection of the Church left me in a spiritual homelessness, disconnected from my spiritual roots. The removal of the heavy robes of patriarchal religion uncovered my rage towards God which I had not previously realised ran so deep. Owning that rage liberated me to come home to an Earth based, feminine, embodied form of spirituality that I had been estranged from.

Imagine what we would feel like if every Sunday we went to a Goddess temple where the holy water, held in a vulvalicious chalice, openly symbolised the life-giving water of the womb and vulva. That the aisle of the temple was the vaginal canal, its red carpet the menses, and the altar the seat of the vulva. That we ritually drank wine as a symbol of woman's life-giving, regenerative menstrual blood (which has been scientifically proven to hold healing stem cells) instead of the blood of a dead man. Notice what you feel in your body as you read this. The symbols adopted by Christianity are rooted in female anatomy and symbology, that were taken under the control of male story writers, for male domination.

The first one to die and be resurrected was her.

The original source of that power and cyclical wisdom still resides in the female body, a fact that 'man' has avidly tried to deny through his biblical propaganda.

Shedding our familial and cultural robes

As children we are born naked into the world of our family and culture that clothes us in norms and expectations. Therefore, Inanna's robes can also be seen to signify the familial and cultural upperworld uniform that Inanna has been cloaked in. The robes are a sign of her belonging, but also, to an extent, her obedience. When we shed this we get to feel, as much as we ever can in a lifetime, who we are without those silent agreements, codes and entrenched expressions. To fall out of belonging with family (whoever family have been for us) and our culture, is big – it literally shakes our roots.

Now to walk away from all this entanglement
that is ours and yet does not belong to us,
that, like the water in an old well,
reflects us trembling and distorts who we are

from "The Departure of the Prodigal Son" by
Rainer Maria Rilke translated by Kim Rosen

Conversely, our familial or personal robes might have been a sign of our rebellion, as much as our conformity. But in the descent, even some of the identities that we have adopted to reject and rebel against upperworld culture will have to be disrobed, so that we can discover who we are when we are stripped of our strongest beliefs and the defence mechanisms that we have adopted to survive. Both conformity and rebellion take energy.

Who are we when we strip ourselves of trying to push for
or against and simply stand naked as we are?

Disobedience is an essential part of Inanna. The moment she chooses to descend, her very existence becomes an embodiment of a different possibility. To become naked is a metaphor for the ways in which we expose and oppose the spirit of the times at an embodied level. It is to become visible, firstly to ourselves, but then to others. If we look right back to Gate One, we discussed how our closest personal relationships are enmeshed in our crowns, they are also entwined with our roots.

Essential disobedience – putting our body and dreams first

One of the things the heroine faces, is the potential and sometimes real loss of those she loves. I spoke to Jacinta Meteur, who at the age of fourteen, fled her village in Kenya alone, to escape Female Genital Mutilation (FGM) and child marriage. Jacinta begins,

> "I think I was fourteen when I left. I didn't tell anyone that I was leaving. But after getting news that you will be cut, you won't go to high school and you have to be married off, I thought 'wow, I don't want to do that, I really want to go to school, I want a career, I have dreams'. So at that point, I had to decide on my own. I had to leave behind something. I had to leave some of my culture, the FGM, the early marriage, I had to leave behind that to be transformed, to be somebody else. I had the information that there was somewhere I could run and be safe and continue my studies. I had to say to myself:

'this is what I want to do and I will do it no matter what'.
So I ran away. In those days it was very difficult for you to get a car.
You had to walk for three or four hours so you could get somewhere
you could get a car and then it was about another four hours to the
city and then another twenty minute walk. And I went alone."

Jacinta had to make the choice to uproot herself from the village, her culture,
her family, from everything she had known, in order to protect her body and
her dreams. She was forced to rescue herself, to become her own heroine. When
I asked Jacinta about the roots of the practice of FGM and the reasons why it
is still practiced, she explained that in Maasai culture it is considered a rite of
passage to womanhood.

"In my culture the idea of FGM is the transition of going between a
child and an adult. So that's why after FGM you get married, because
they believe at that point, now you have become a woman, you can
have children, you can stay with a husband, cook for a husband...
That is the main purpose of FGM in Maasai culture, that when
you have gone through FGM you are a woman. And secondly, they
believe that when you get a cut, it will be easier for you to give birth.
When you are not cut, people don't want to be near you when you
deliver a child. They say, 'I can't help her because she is not cut'. And
sometimes, they do it when women are giving birth, sometimes they
just force cut you when you are delivering a baby. Because otherwise
they believe you are still a child, that you are not yet a woman, that
you are not mature, if you have not gone through the cut. They think
that you are dirty – it's really a lot."

In reality, the scar tissue created by FGM makes childbirth much more dangerous, putting both mothers and babies at higher risk. Babies often get stuck
on the way out of a vaginal canal that is restricted by scar tissue, consequently,
the incidence of brain damage is high in these communities. It is painfully ironic
to me that the initiation into womanhood requires girls to sacrifice their most
intimate anatomy and capacity for sexual pleasure. To cut a woman's root is to
try to sever her connection with her power and make her obedient and docile.

This is an extreme, barbaric example of the way that women's bodies are owned and abused in patriarchal culture. As women we are all too commonly forced to choose between accommodating the culture, or being true to ourselves. Somalian born, Hibo Wardere is a survivor of FGM and in her powerful book, *Cut*, she states,

In some cultures, to be a woman is to be condemned to a lifetime of pain. To be a woman means subjection to child abuse, to ensure that your 'virtue' remains intact, that your sexuality is controlled and that you are accepted by your community. Unfortunately, by chance, I was born into one of those cultures – just like 60,000 other girls in Britain. FGM is a British problem. FGM is a global problem.

In the UK it is estimated that 137,000 women are affected by FGM[*]. But what happens at the roots of the body and family is often hidden, private, not spoken about, exiled, like Ereshkigal. This makes abuse, in whatever form it manifests, much more likely to remain hidden. If a girl is not educated about her body, if she does not have names for it, if it is not spoken about, then it will be much more difficult for her to articulate her experiences, which is a form of disempowerment. This gate asks us to uproot what has been held in silence. To dare to challenge cultural norms and practices that oppress us and deny who we are. The roots of communities and culture are upheld by a certain amount of necessary social conformity. But since patriarchal dominator societies are actually rooted in the exploitation and oppression of women, it means that by simply re-entering our bodies as our own, we break the social codes of the upperworld and consequently, disrupt any social bonds that perpetuate our oppression. This can impact our closest relationships. As Jacinta explores,

"The big part is not doing what your parents wanted you to do, because they feel like you are now disobedient, you don't respect them, because what they are doing, you refuse to do that. And now you moved to be somebody else, to create a different kind of culture for yourself. Because now whatever you see them doing, it's not what you believe in and it's not right to your eyes. What they raised you to do and be, you are doing the opposite of that. To me the decision was

[*]   Source: July 2014 report released by City University London and Equality Now

clear, the only thing was that I felt I had betrayed my people. People you love, that have been with you, they have raised you, you know, so sometimes it feels like there is a betrayal that you have done."

What does it mean when the people we love, the culture we want to belong to, is incompatible with our desires, needs, bodies? What does it mean when we can no longer sacrifice ourselves to fit in? When Jacinta chose to leave her village, like Inanna she chose to descend, to go into the wilderness and forage for a *different culture* for herself. To support herself, she did what the heroine does, she looked for a Ninshubur to bang the drum for her and in this case give her refuge. The place that Jacinta had heard about was the V-Day Safe House founded by Agnes Pareyio and the Tasaru Ntomonok Initiative, a woman-led community organisation working to end child marriage and FGM. Agnes Pareyio is a survivor of FGM herself. At fourteen she was cut, even though she had protested against it, social pressure made her submit. Afterwards, she vowed,

I promised myself, on the day my vagina was mutilated, that I would never let another girl be mutilated.

For many years Agnes Pareyio worked slowly and steadfastly on foot, going from village to village in Kenya, educating people about the dangers of FGM. Then in 2002 she met V (formerly Eve Ensler) whose organisation, V-Day Org, together with the Tasaru Ntomonok Initiative, helped set-up the V-Day Safe House. Twenty years on, the Safe House still gives refuge to girls fleeing FGM and child marriage. This was the house that Jacinta fled to.

Facing and feeling the impact of abuse

When we become naked, we begin to see not only ourselves differently, but also the culture. As with all of the gates, we begin to realise that some of what has been normal for us, is actually not normal at all, and is sometimes even abusive. Abuse affects our relationships with our roots. When we experience abuse our energy is forced up into the higher centres of the body as a way of surviving the unpleasant experiences happening to us – we dissociate, as we talked about in Chapter Three. Patterns of dissociation are painful because they keep us fragmented and disembodied. Therefore, acknowledging any trauma and abuse we have experienced is a vital part of the descent back down to our roots. But to admit abuse can be threatening to our sense of self and our relationships.

In Hibo Wardere's book, she speaks about the girls who have been cut when they were babies, or too young to remember. Some of these women grow up thinking that their vulva has always been this way, that it is natural for it to take fifteen minutes to pee, for sex to be acutely painful: they believe that this is just what being a woman feels like. Some women only discover that they have been mutilated when they give birth in a Western hospital and it is referenced by the medical staff taking care of them. This can cause significant psychological distress, as women realise that the people they love and trusted actually mutilated their body without their consent. When Inanna is disrobed, she is asked to enter a new relationship with her body, including any abuses and traumas. Then she can begin to feel and comprehend the way that these experiences have shaped her relationship with herself and her world.

Though FGM is an extreme example of bodily abuse, there are plenty of other ways that abusive social control plays out on women's bodies. As social animals we want to be accepted and so we all, to greater or lesser degrees, try to shape our bodies to make them socially acceptable. This can result in self-sacrificing or self-injuring behaviours such as: constant dieting, body dysmorphia, anorexia, bulimia, plastic surgery or botox, or being in abusive relationships. It can also be more subtle, like the denial of our own desires, hatred/fear of our femininity, putting ourselves in dangerous sexual situations, or overworking and the inability to rest. Additionally, the increased popularity and availability of porn is having a significant impact on human sexual relationships and how people perceive the body. Many porn stars have had labiaplasties, where the labia are cut to a 'neater', more uniform, shape. This gives people a false idea of what women's vulvas actually look like. There are many women now choosing to cut themselves by having labiaplasties, which is said to be the world's fastest growing cosmetic procedure[*]. Women can be held captive by a very narrow view of what being female 'should' be and look like. This can lead women to reject their own bodies and sex, or conversely, women get caught in a perpetual struggle to measure up to impossible beauty ideals, striving to be more 'womanly' – what-

[*] Source: article in *The Independent* newspaper: independent.co.uk/news/health/labiaplasty-vagina-surgery-cosmetic-procedure-plastic-study-international-society-aesthetic-plastic-surgeons-usa-a7837181.html

ever that means. In the midst of these upperworld dogmas, we can lose ourselves entirely.

To de-robe is to take off some of these societal distortions and expectations. So that we can ask,

If I am not confined by ideas about what I should look
and feel like, who am I? And how do I feel?

Gender-diverse people and men may also go through this sloughing off of confining gender norms. The descent as a journey into partnership is about creating more and more diversity. I believe this gate is a call home to our own unique nature and an awakening to the ways that the cultural robes have robbed us of relationship with that.

The Sky God (Emperor) is wearing no clothes

As we reveal ourselves, we also see our environment and community in a whole new light. To be naked is to see more clearly. You probably know the old Hans Christian Anderson story of *The Emperor's New Clothes*. It is about a vain Emperor, or for our purposes let's say a Sky God, who is obsessed with his appearance and having many fine clothes. Two trickster weavers decide to exploit his vanity in order to dupe him. They promise that they will weave him the finest clothes. They tell him that the wonderful fabric will remain invisible to anyone unfit to be in power. Eager not to fall from power, the Sky God pretends to see the robes, and even when the weavers work with invisible looms, he does not admit that he cannot see the fabric. When finished, the Sky God puts on the imaginary clothes and goes out naked on a parade through the streets to show off his exquisite attire. His courtiers go along with the façade and carry his false robes, along with all his subjects, who celebrate and compliment him on his fabulous outfit. Only a girl in the crowd pipes up to say,

"But the Sky God is wearing no clothes!"

The innocence of our wisdom is what we return to in the admission of our own nakedness: a momentary freedom from the cultural politenesses that have schooled us out of saying what is in front of us.

Gate Seven asks us to admit what we see, rather than deny or distort it (at first if only to ourselves). The story of *The Emperor's New Clothes* is testament to the power of community cohesion, whose shadow can tip us into collusion with ignorance and even blatant abuse. The energy of the naked feminine is a powerful antidote to this.

The heroine as an embodied agent of change

Once the robes are removed it becomes much more difficult to deny the reality of our experiences. Old personal and cultural identities die and are transformed, which changes the shape of our root systems. For a time, we may feel an acute sense of homelessness as we are stripped of the clothing that has covered us since birth. Returning to Jacinta's story, she spoke to this,

> "When I look back at the culture, the community, I see many things which are not right to me. And sometimes I feel like some things are not true, because you reach a point where you think: are these things happening really? Because they are too strong. I came out of them, I don't believe in them anymore. You feel like they are too strange, that this can't be happening right now. But it is.
> Culture is so instilled in us, so we believe in it, it really takes a lot to transform that person to believe that there is something more out there than what they believe in. But now I have this power to help to transform others. Now that I really understand what is happening in my culture, my work – which is very hard – is to help make change. It cannot be done overnight. This needs to be done, slowly, slowly, slowly. So that when you transform two, the two can transform others and keep doing that."

Jacinta points to the transformative effects of the heroine's journey and the powerful waves that it creates in communities. Agnes Pareyio, Hibo Wardere and Jacinta Meteur have common ground, in that through their rising and rejection of the practice FGM, they have become embodied agents of change. The base chakra holds the energy of our tribal roots, therefore, when we step through Gate Seven into deeper grounding in ourselves, we begin to make change simply by being more and more of who we are. This is the leadership of the heroine. Being naked is a metaphor for being visible. We need visible heroines to create new stories, new possibilities, maps for those girls following behind us. This is how we create woman-honouring lineages, a her-story that can be a companion and guide for us as we traverse the unknowns of the underworld and the sometimes very lonely and frightening territory of confronting what we can no longer live by. As Pareyio highlights,

When women stand up and defend themselves, it works. In 1975, 98% of women were mutilated just like I was. Today, it is 27%. That's 27% too many, but it's also the sign of a revolution. It wasn't handed down on high. It was fought for by me and my sisters. I believe that no woman should call herself free until all women are free.

What I respect about Agnes Pareyio's approach is that she seeks to mediate between girls and their families and communities. The V-Day Safe House has fostered a grassroots, collaborative partnership approach and it is working. As Pareyio says, *it wasn't handed down on high.* It is not decreed by the Sky Gods. Instead it is about helping people understand that there is another option and the reasons why those options are of benefit, not only to the girls, but to their whole community. What is good for women is actually good for everyone. This approach does not seek to exile anyone, or repeat oppression. Instead, like Inanna when she goes to meet Ereshkigal, it is about relationship, sisterhood and power with, not over, others.

Jacinta now works for the S.H.E. College Fund founded by Kim Rosen. S.H.E. supports girls after they leave safe houses in the Narok County where Jacinta grew up, to go onto a college education. Jacinta told me about their work,

"Now we have forty women and ten who have already graduated and almost 70% have got jobs. It's amazing and it really gives us the motivation to go beyond what we think we can do. Because you find that often the girls are the only ones in their family who have reached university or who have got diploma courses or vocational training and now their family are looking up to them. Because they are beginning to see that once girls graduate and get a job, they can support their family and the whole village can see that. The narratives are changing, because if you look at the students who have finished, then the parents are now trying to educate their younger sisters."

As Jacinta and the young women she supports show, by daring to disrobe old confining cultural ideas about what girls can be and do, they are changing the landscape of Kenyan culture.

This is the final gate to the underworld, it is dark and mysterious and the path is not always clear, so, like Jacinta says, it has to happen slowly. This is especially important when working with trauma. If the body has not been a safe place to be, if we just land straight into Gate Seven we will likely feel so overwhelmed that we will check out of the body again. The seven gates provide a staged (not always sequential) re-entry into the body and our unprocessed material. This doesn't mean it is not challenging and uncomfortable. But the descent operates at the slow time of the underworld which gives us time to titrate our experience and learn to tolerate more and more feeling. The slowness may be confronting in itself, especially if being hyper and always on the go has been the way we have avoided ourselves. But regardless, *"the underworld has its own rules, they may not be questioned"*.

This gate calls on us to reveal what has not yet been revealed. Community and cultural change happens in the bodies of those who create that culture first. So at Gate Seven, we enter the absolute depths of the depths. Where we must feel, listen, pray and grieve. As we do so, we put tendrils into the Earth and seek out connections that will feed and nourish us. I believe this is how we change the world from the ground up.

The heroine is one who is looking for another way inside her own body and life, and in doing so she might furrow a path for others. When women rise rooted we can support each other, but first we must disrobe. The robes are the compost that help fertilise the new soil from which we will grow.

Becoming naked – an embodied practice

Stand in front of a full-length mirror naked (if that feels too confronting then don't override that feeling and instead take as much clothing off as feels okay for you in this moment, you can revisit this practice as many times as you need).

Take time to look at your own body, you can also explore with touch if it feels right and notice what you feel. There may be lots of feelings and thoughts, or not a lot. Notice what/if any feelings of judgement, pleasure, rejection, pain, love, numbness arrive in the witnessing of your naked body. Breathe. Feel. Call in your inner Ninshubur to behold you.

Then perhaps put some music on, or not, whatever you prefer. And begin to move from inside the body. If you find it hard to move from the inside, try closing your eyes, to feel in rather than move from looking on the outside. Feel the air moving against your naked body. Wake up your own sensuality. Feel free to touch your body and skin. Invite your own nakedness and see what is revealed to you.

THE UNDERWORLD

Naked and bowed low, Inanna entered the throne room...
Ereshkigal fastened on Inanna they eye of death.
She spoke against her the word of wrath.
She uttered against her the cry of death.
She struck her.
Inanna was turned into a corpse,
A piece of rotting meat,
And was hung from a hook on the wall.

Diane Wolkstein and Samuel Kramer,
Inanna: Queen of Heaven and Earth

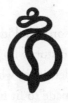

Chapter 8

INANNA'S DEATH

Inanna descends in search of sisterhood, but at the crescendo of the descent, when the sisters finally meet, Ereshkigal kills Inanna. All that is left is a rotting piece of meat on a hook: such a visceral image. This is woman initiating woman. Woman initiated by her own dark material within the crucible of her life. In this moment, Ereshkigal is the war-mongerer, the devourer, the destroyer *and* she is the victim, the oppressed and the ostracised. In this act of killing Inanna are so many layers. When Ereshkigal stakes Inanna, she initiates herself and Inanna into a death marriage of the complex energies of the masculine and feminine. Why a death marriage?

Because the separation, the split, has to die.

Through this initiation, the personas and identities that have been put on top of Inanna as the Sky Queen, that distort who she is, can finally die. These could be called her 'false self' or 'false identities', which are all the personas, roles and unhealthy compromises she has made to fit into her personal relationships and the culture. Moving from Queen to being naked and bowed low, is a descent from her mind's dominance and control, back into full partnership with her body and the ripening consciousness within her: not through dominance but through submission.

The body is a wild thing, a feral thing and a vulnerable thing. When she meets the Death Goddess she also meets her own powerlessness and exhaustion. Now we have to admit our life as it is, which in this moment is far from what we hoped for or expected. In this death we lose all hope for another solution, or the ability to pursue anything that might look like a tidy outcome. We must yield and submit.

To face our lack of control elicits a radical shift within our being. Physically, in my experience, at this point something inside me just gave up. Through the gates, when Inanna keeps asking the question *"what is this?"* there is some sense of hope, questioning, fight even. But when she is staked, the questions end.

It is human nature to hang on for as long as possible, because these identities feel like such a fundamental part of who we believe ourselves to be – an idea that is reinforced by modern cultural ideals. When we are asked to surrender, it seems such an absurd and alien path. This final submission is the death of all fight. Now naked, even the hope that it can be another way must die.

Giving Up Hope – Meeting Death

When we actually meet this rock face in our own life story, the reality of it is bleak. For months, I felt like a walking zombie. I dropped the kids at school, I was still doing my life, and was grateful for my life, but some other part of me was utterly broken in a way that I can hardly articulate. On one of the worst days, my husband was working away and the kids were at school and for just a few hours I completely gave in. I didn't have to pretend for anyone. I got into bed, curled into a ball and felt like I would never get up again. A huge part of myself, that I had relied on to keep me going, had gone and I could make no sense of it. I felt as though I didn't know how to do life any other way. It felt impossible. And yet, bizarrely, I was still doing life. The Ninshubur part of me was holding the structure of mother and wife together for my family, and even teacher for my students. But another part was in pieces, deconstructed and scattered. Lucy H. Pearce gave voice to her experience of this place,

"Just before I was diagnosed as autistic and we were in the absolute eye of the storm, I just couldn't do it anymore. It was, 'I cannot live anymore'. It was, 'I am dying. This is actually it. There is nothing more

I can give or do.' I felt like a dead person walking. I was in our packing room, trying to pack an order and I just curled up in a ball on the floor and said, 'This is it.' I have gone through anxiety, depression, suicidal thoughts, but this was different. This was like: this flesh and this soul cannot endure anything else, not even another breath. Just being in a foetal position knowing that you can't get up, you can't think another thought. I had that twice in this process where all I could do was just curl up. I felt that I couldn't live anymore, not through despair, but complete exhaustion. The life impulse was just gone.

To me when you say Inanna, that's what I feel. There is nowhere to go. You can't go up, you can't go down, you can't go left, you can't go right, you're not really alive, and yet…here you are. It's not even the most scary place to be, there are many scarier places I have been in my head. But it was the closest I have been to death. My heart was beating, my lungs were working but I was dead. And then you get up and you have to carry on somehow. You are in the underworld, 100% dead, and yet you're having to pretend that you're not. It was like a chord snapped, an energetic chord snapped to what I would call my hopeful self, my idealist or utopian self. And that went – hope went."

At the deepest depths of the underworld what I believe we meet is necessary hopelessness. There are many tales that warn that too much soul can drive you mad, and if we do not find the help we need to release us from the hook, psychosis or enduring depression can ensue. When our upperworld identity hangs on the stake, it is unclear how, when, or if, we will ever be released. Linda Hartley explores,

> When we embark upon this journey of descent, we enter the place of deepest depression, yet it is rare for suicides to occur when we fall to this depth. We are already dead, so death can be no escape – it cannot even be considered a possibility. In the depths of the descent, there is neither the will nor the energy for even this act. This is an unimaginable place to one who has not experienced it.

Yet for me, in this impossible darkness, was still a sense of something sacred at work. On some bone deep level, it was the feeling that something was shaping me, in a way that only Ereshkigal could. The myth was an essential Ninshubur in the depths. When I spoke to Sophie Jane Hardy, she articulated something similar in her own experience,

> "Eventually, I did the counting out of pills. We had lots of pills in the house because Ade had had a back operation. I got them all out and googled what you need to take an overdose. I was serious about it. But then found out that there wasn't enough and I came to. But I reached the point of thinking that if this isn't possible, then death is the only answer. Because I can't bear to have this longing and not have it met. This is why things like the Inanna myth started to make more sense to me, because the myth was big enough to hold the size of the grief I was experiencing."

What is common to all the stories in this book is the magnitude of the forces at work. They are incomprehensible and yet real and so powerful. The underworld energies suspend you in death, within a life that is somehow still moving. In longing that cannot be met, that stretches us to endure feelings beyond what we could have imagined before. It is mythic in proportion and it sits right in the midst of the day-to-day of the supermarket, work and all that is normal in life.

> *What we choose to fight is so tiny!*
> *What fights us is so great!*
> *If only we would let ourselves be dominated*
> *as things do by some immense storm,*
> *we would become strong too, and not need names.*
> *When we win it's with small things,*
> *and the triumph itself makes us small.*
> *What is extraordinary and eternal*
> *does not want to be bent by us.*

from "The Man Watching" by Rilke, translated by Robert Bly

As my old identities finally died, so too did many of my old judgements, defences and my self-righteousness. The war inside me ended in a significant way – there was a relief in that. Ereshkigal's rage is righteous and its shadow is the destructive part of each one of us: the one inside us who wants to hurt others, our own cruelty. Until we get to know these darker flavours of our being we cannot take responsibility for them.

When Inanna, as the light of our consciousness, submits, she admits her own darkness. She comes face-to-face and is slain by the witnessing of her own destruction and her own perpetration. Often for women (not always), that has most prominently shown up as perpetration towards self: eating disorders, patterns of self-abandonment, self-injuring behaviours are all forms of self-harm and cruelty. It can and does also include the ways we have harmed others.

Personally, where I had previously seen myself purely as the victim of toxic masculinity, when I was impaled by Ereshkigal, I woke up to how my own shadow had played into the dynamics. How I had relied on certain males, and women with a strong masculine energy for power and praise, to avoid the more frightening route of fully embodying my own power and work. And how I had sometimes subconsciously avoided relationships of equality with other women for fear of rejection. I also became starkly aware of how harshly I had judged others, and myself. Without the armour of my victimhood or superiority, all that was left was grief and a sort of inertia. I no longer identified with what I was before, but what I was becoming was not yet clear either.

It is incredibly humbling to witness our own darkness, and so life enriching. Once we stop trying to exile Ereshkigal, the life energy that has been held hostage can finally start to be freed. Angela Farmer spoke to me about her experience of this part of the descent,

"I love that aspect of 'total annihilation'. In the early days, when I shared this myth with students, they looked a little shocked when I told them that this is the part I really love! The Greek myth of Persephone describes her yearly descent to the underworld, but she does not die. Inanna is annihilated. There is nothing left of her, just a bit of flesh, hung up on a meat hook. I find that cleansing and total. Other stories fade in comparison. This, for me, was 100% yes! Reality. That's it. To finally drop into that sense of 'there's nothing left of me' opens the door to healing from the depths."

There is a cleansing, a release, that happens when we let die that which we are most afraid of losing. And a liberation in dissolving so much of what we have called "I". When we let go of our names, will power, stories, roles, ideas…who are we then? This death is the death of our personal shaped hope, the death of the stories we thought defined us and importantly, the death of our attachment to bending the outcome to our own will. Constantly trying to bend things to our own will is exhausting. As Rilke says, *what is extraordinary and eternal does not want to be bent by us.* Ereshkigal shapes us, not the other way around. As spiritual teacher and author Gangaji names,

> *Hope itself is some projection of a me, into a future, in order to avoid the catastrophe that is sensed in the present. Whether it is sensed through a newspaper or the television, or just the sensations in one's body. It is not for the faint of heart, it is not a mass teaching, it is not a cult teaching. Mass teachings and cult teachings give you hope. It is a willingness to stand alone where you are and face what you are most afraid of facing – the annihilation of you, without any hope of survival... The end of your life as you know it. The end of you as you think yourself. The end of all that you have accumulated or gained, or lost, the end of it – period.*

Giving up hope is an incredibly foreign concept within a culture that constantly strives for perpetual youth and the avoidance of death at all costs. Historically, we had a much more intimate relationship with death. Our life expectancy was lower, and it would have been normal for a family to lose at least one child. Our medical advancements have changed this. In England, in the past, we would have laid our dead out in the family home and people would have come to pay their respects. Today, tending to the dead is most often carried out through the funeral home, rather than by family. We live an all-round more sanitised existence which can leave us estranged from the palpable edge of mystery where life and death meet.

Like Ereshkigal, death has been pushed to the margins of our society. This means that when we meet with death we don't know how to be in relationship with it, or how to behold another as they move towards their own death. What I noticed when walking towards death alongside my grandma, was that until the final twelve hours, the emphasis was on keeping her alive, rather than holding her as she moved towards death. And that's understandable. Her deterioration happened quite quickly and I think I expected her to bounce back. But also it was something to do with my relationship with death, which at the time I viewed as something to stave off rather than accept and hold. Through that experience, I learned that the best thing we can offer someone who is dying is the willingness to be present with what is unfolding.

Death is a portal into the depths, and if we cannot slow to its tempo, we miss its gifts. Deaths and births are not times to rush. There is a strange vitality in death, a special suspension in magic that we miss when we lose contact with death itself. On the days when some of the most treasured people in my life have died, alongside the grief, I have also felt suspended in an alternate reality, where even amidst my sadness the magic of life shines brighter. If we do not keep death near, we do not treasure life as fully as we ought. In his book, "The Five Invitations", Buddhist teacher and author Frank Ostaseski explains,

> Life and death are a package deal. You cannot pull them apart. In Japanese zen, the term shoji translates to 'birth-death'. There is no separation between life and death other than a small hyphen, a thin line that connects the two. We cannot truly be alive without maintaining an awareness of death. Death is not waiting for us at the end of a long road. Death is always with us, in the marrow of every passing moment. She is the secret teacher hiding in plain sight. She helps us discover what matters most.

Journalling enquiry into your relationship with death

1. Take a moment to feel what is dying in your life right now. It could be the physical death of a loved one, or your own death, death of a role, job, a relationship or menopause, to name a few.

2. Write about how you feel in relationship to this death: withdrawn, keeping busy, checking out, comfort eating, calm, liberated? See what shows up.

3. How can you call death closer to you in this process? What lessons are emerging from this ending?

To press death back to the margins is another way to deny nature. At one time, the oldest person in the family would have been the wisdom keeper. We now live in a society that praises youth. People still travel to the other side of the world to sit in the darshan of someone who embodies the depths. Yet we ship our elders off to the lazy chair and pay them little attention. We are living in a world with an increasing ageing population, yet sparsely populated with true elders. Elders are ones who have been seasoned by life experience and have been initiated, which can happen at any age. We are an immature society and sadly this means that few people walk the path of becoming an elder.

Working as a therapist, I find time and again that endings hold some of the most fertile moments of the whole therapeutic process, because when we meet death, all our hidden coping strategies and vulnerabilities come up to be seen and felt. Death disarms us and deepens our sensitivity to life. Yet, I feel that fear of the dark feminine is part of a healthy reverence for death. After all, her entrance into our lives can take away people we love and things we had hoped for. Ultimately, the path we are all destined for is surrender. Even if we go out fighting, death will make us submit in the end, as Inanna does when Ereshkigal impales her.

Chapter 9

MEETING ERESHKIGAL – RECLAIMING OUR SACRED RAGE

In the face of Inanna, all Ereshkigal's rage rises up. She stakes Inanna with a meat hook and hangs her as a corpse to rot.

The raw power of Ereshkigal to take life, is exactly the devouring qualities of the feminine that patriarchy has worked so hard to keep at bay. She is the fierce, carnal power of the dark feminine. So it is not a total surprise that this potency is exactly what women are socialised to disown inside of ourselves. Rage is often one of the dismembered expressions of women, to our detriment.

Ereshkigal is the embodiment of our wild, untamed, sacred rage. She holds the rage of all the raped, exiled, oppressed women and the abused Earth. She is the vital disobedience held within our *eros*, the growls and snarls that emerge from the roots of our roots, the bared teeth, the refusal to be nice and placate. She is Durga riding the wild tiger between her legs, she the mama bear, the wild shriek of the banshee, the cackle of Baba Yaga, the power of Lilith and the holy chthonic power of Pachamama. She is the dark veil of night and the uncompromising softness of change. She is the embodiment of our unswerving loyalty to what is here, right now, even if that is terrifying.

She is needed if we ever want to be fully alive.

I feel it is so poignant that Ereshkigal is a goddess of ancient Sumer, where his-storically women have been abused on such a massive scale. As Iraqi artist and writer, Tamara Albanna illuminates,

When Al-Qaeda came into towns and raped women and girls en-masse, we descended. When Daesh swept through the land, and raped and murdered women and girls – while the world watched – we descended further and further. Wars and sanctions, starvation and hopelessness – all by the patriarchal machine – we descended.

Anger is often regarded as a harmful or undesirable quality in a woman but, without the expression of anger, a part of our essential life force is cut off, making many women forget that when someone is not very nice to us (or worse) that we are within our rights to say *"that is not okay"*. We need anger to live in integrity, without it we can become passive, unboundaried and disenfranchised from our own authority. Only when we admit our rage can we relearn to express it, rooted in the understanding that it is a feeling as valuable and necessary as any other.

Every woman has a well-stocked arsenal of anger potentially useful against those oppressions, personal and institutional, which brought that anger into being. Focused with precision it can become a powerful source of energy serving progress and change. And when I speak of change, I do not mean a simple switch of positions or a temporary lessening of tensions, nor the ability to smile or feel good. I am speaking of a basic and radical alteration in those assumptions underlining our lives.

Audre Lorde, *The Uses of Anger: Women Responding to Racism*

The heroine is one who makes a commitment to the process of composting the *assumptions* that underlie our lives. A commitment to uncover and take responsibility for our biases, privilege, oppression and ignorance and then endeavour to move with greater awareness inside and out. Because oppression isn't only something that is enacted from the outside onto us, but it is internalized into our systems in all sorts of intricate ways.

We embody oppression.

Ereshkigal's exile *is* the embodiment of our own oppression. Therefore, an unequivocal requirement of the descent is that we change the *assumptions* that

Lorde names, at an embodied level of our being. The heroine may affect change externally, but the primary shifts happen in her being and body first. I feel an essential aspect of what Ereshkigal puts to death, in herself and in Inanna, is ignorance.

An enquiry around rage and anger

What is your relationship with anger?

How do you show it?

How do you hide/suppress it?

What does your angry voice sound like?

When you were younger how were you encouraged or discouraged to express anger?

Notice what you feel in your body as you explore this. If it helps journal about it.

Reclaiming our Inner Predator

The feminine is so often associated with the yin qualities of softness, surrender and receptivity, but another facet of the feminine is ferocity. Motherhood is an initiation into the fullness of feminine power. A fundamental part of that is the fierce feminine who will show up with a violent "no!" if she has to. She who will risk everything, including her own life, for the sake of her young. This is the face of the feminine that I feel we need more of in our world. And let's be clear, it is not exclusively available to mothers, it lives in all women.

I call this the yang feminine, yang being the active principle predominantly associated with the masculine, but that is very much present in the feminine as well. If you think of the symbol of the yin yang, both the yin side and the yang side hold a circle of the other aspect. We all have yin and yang aspects regardless of sex. For males to embrace their yin qualities and females to embrace their yang is a part of the journey to maturity. When the yang feminine is denied, it amputates essential aspects of our energy, psyche, expression and what Kimberly Ann Johnson calls our "healthy aggression", as seen in the fierce lioness defending her young. But when a woman expresses this more ferocious side of her being she is commonly berated for it and, like Ereshkigal, is sent back to the underworld.

As women, I believe one of the key reasons that we descend is to reclaim, remember and reconnect with our inner predator. If we go back to the Inanna-Ereshkigal myth as a map of trauma integration, once we have thawed our freeze and learned how to down-regulate our nervous systems, then we must also remember how to up-regulate into our *healthy aggression*. All of the rage that we did not or could not express has a vitality inside it. Rage doesn't go away. Like a wolf she will keep scratching at the door until we admit her. If we cannot allow and express our rage, it will be like a dark shadow that we have to work increasingly hard to keep at bay. Holding the door shut to rage is hard work and zaps our energy. Imagine the wild wolf at the door and you pushing back with all your might, whilst trying to remain calm – it's exhausting and futile.

For years, I associated yang energy with perpetration and subconsciously disowned it. We need to reclaim Ereshkigal's integrity and her assertive wild nature. This is what Kimberly Ann Johnson refers to as "activating your inner predator" she suggests that,

Restoring the predator side of our system is about coming into contact with our natural impulses of self-protection and self-defence, trusting that those will kick in if and when we need them. It's about getting out of freeze in order to create something new, so that your default response to threat doesn't have to be prey...in other words, our need to protect ourselves becomes greater than our concerns about making too much noise, being nice, disappointing someone, or being a 'bad patient' or a 'bad daughter' or 'needy girlfriend', or whatever role you may feel compelled to fill. This ferocity is an embodiment of self-love and unquestioned self-worth.

Ereshkigal's stake is an initiation into our own ferocity, a penetration of the one in us who is so concerned about how we will be perceived and what others will think. For a woman to own her penetrative energy is to stand up in her power. In doing so, she actually interrupts patterns of unhealthy accommodation.

Though our fear of rage may be acute (be that our own rage or the rage of others), the irony is that without owning this predatory energy we cannot protect ourselves and are more likely to be preyed upon. I want to emphasise here, that accommodation is one of women's superpowers, and is a good survival strategy, especially if we have had abusers who are big and threatening to us. But when *prey* becomes our default position, in all situations, we lose contact with healthy boundaries. If repeated enough, we lose our ability to even hear our body's "no" anymore.

As a culture we've not permitted women to show sympathetic fight responses, and as a result we are often not well practiced in them. What that means is that we don't always look angry when we are angry. That's a problem.

Kimberly Ann Johnson, *Call of the Wild*

The fight response comes from our sympathetic nervous system, the part that primes our bodies for action. Johnson suggests that these instinctive defences to dangerous or stressful situations have been kerbed. The good news is, if we recognise this pattern inside ourselves, we can then begin to actively re-engage and reclaim our predatory responses. For those of us whose inner predator has been muted, reclaiming Ereshkigal's sacred animal rage can be an incredibly enlivening and vibrant part of the ascent.

We can be humbled by our anger: its aliveness is both exciting and terrible. Never having shown much anger in my life, I remember being pushed to the edge in the way that only children, or a very close relationship to someone you are a carer for, can push you. I was exhausted and it was the end of a long day with two children under three. My husband was away, my eldest daughter wouldn't get into bed and all of a sudden this surge of rage came out of me, "Get into your bed!" the voice shouted. It was my voice, but not one that even I was very familiar with.

My daughter heard Ereshkigal in my voice because the response was immediate. She got into bed and said, *"Mummy you're scaring me"*. Those words melted me and within moments a tear slipped from my eye and I was able to hold her, apologise and repair it. This is not an episode I am proud of, and in fact for months afterwards I carried shame about it. But as I retell it now, I can say that it was not a bad thing. Our children need to see our rage: that's how they know it is an acceptable emotion. Rage is an essential aspect of feeling our boundaries and self-protection. Obviously if we are constantly scaring our children, we need to seek some help, but my daughter got to feel the energy of rage and with it, my boundary.

Our rage has a life force, it is an energy that when disowned can act out in very painful ways. But when we can own it and become more intimate with its flavours, it has the power to make positive change in us, and that is key here.

We often enact anger in the hope of changing the other, but the most important thing our anger can change is ourselves.

When we take responsibility for what is alive in us, it can reveal itself to us. Like Inanna, it becomes naked and unveiled. Then we can get to know it and perhaps even in the right circumstances, feel the pleasure of its release.

When we haven't been in contact with our inner predator for many years, if ever, then when we begin to reclaim this aspect of ourselves we will inevitably 'get it wrong'. Or if we have been stuck in rage as our default, then our journey may be to soften the fight and feel the vulnerability underneath that. Whichever way round it configures in you, whatever is emerging out of the dark of our subconscious will take time to mature inside of us. This is not a reason to shy away from it, on the contrary, it is a reason to go towards it. It is another great humbler. Getting it 'wrong' means we get the opportunity to say, *"I made a mistake, I'm sorry"*. This is one of the greatest spiritual practices I know. This is also one very simple way of bringing our spiritual practice into the grounding of our daily life. To this day, when my rage acts out, I find it so hard to say sorry. I have to get over myself, to find the humility enough to make a sincere apology and I still don't always manage it. What I am referring to here is not a self-flagellating apology doused in the need for approval of the other, that is another defence mechanism. But rather, a genuine admission that I got it wrong. When we 'get it wrong' can we be humble enough to learn, to own it, rather than try to cover it? Can we become more naked day-to-day?

Meeting the Shadow of Our Anger – Perpetration and Victimhood

The enactment of Ereshkigal's wrath on Inanna sheds light on what has previously been hidden. In my experience, it is a potent and deeply humbling process when the rageful or violent one within us acts out and we actually get to witness our own cruelty. From this point of view, staking Inanna is also a moment of conscious awakening for Ereshkigal, which initiates the birthing of new awareness within her.

If we do not submit to Ereshkigal's rage and allow its expression, then that energy does not go away. What we do not express will usually find another way out, and if it can't do it in the light, it will find a way to do it in the dark. This could be in the form of illness, disruptions/pain in our menstrual cycle or self-harming behaviours, toxic relationships, unhealthy relational dynamics and, at worst, openly vindictive or abusive behaviour that hurts others.

Ereshkigal is Inanna's shadow and the part of the feminine that will destroy indiscriminately. She is what 'man' most fears that he will be consumed by. If we do not know and claim her power, she can show up as toxic femininity, which can be equally as manipulative and destructive as the toxic masculine. When we are hurt, in retaliation, we can become vengeful. Vengeance has an entirely different feel to sacred rage. The shadow of Ereshkigal's rageful action towards Inanna is the lashing out that is enacted by the wounded parts of us, that we do not take responsibility for. We use vengeance to get back at others, the problem is that we have to exile something to do it – our pain. The potency of our vengeance intoxicates us and drowns out our feelings of vulnerability. In doing so it not only detaches us from *feeling* our pain, but also the pain that we cause to the other. Ironically, from our victimhood, we then become the perpetrator.

Ereshkigal cannot welcome Inanna into the underworld because she blames her for her oppression. Ironically, casting ourselves as the perpetual victim is another survival strategy. Embracing the ways we have been victimised and tending to our wounding can be a vital part of the descent. But if our victimhood becomes a fixed identity it can prevent our growth and hold us in purgatory.

The split between victim and perpetrator can keep us in the underworld. I am not saying that we need to heal the rift with those who hurt or abused us. We might, but it is not a given. For me the primary focus is on how we have inter-nalised Inanna and Ereshkigal, the victim and perpetrator within. How they are relating inside of us?

The way out of the split is to feel our pain.

When the heroine crosses the threshold of the underworld, she must admit the hurt others have caused her, and the hurt she has caused to both herself and others. Then we can tend to the victim within ourselves *and* we can get to know our own violence, and come into a more intimate relationship with our darkness.

The Fierce Feminine

Collectively, we need the fierce feminine to call out the abuses in the world and of the planet. In current times, the oppressed fierce feminine is finding destruc-tive ways to express herself. I believe we see this in the more extreme weather conditions we are experiencing: the burning Arctic, the wars that rage through our world and the melting of the polar ice caps. The feminine is screaming to be heard and it is beyond time that we started to listen. In order to enter into new relationship with our feminine in all her facets, we have to stop being daughters of the patriarchy and begin to embrace our authority from a different ground. This ground has been grossly under-populated and therefore can feel very un-familiar (in the literal sense of the word un-familied), unstable and frightening. It requires a death to happen inside of us. As Queen of the Underworld, Eresh-kigal's rage holds the laws of the descent in place. It is the demanding part of Ereshkigal that commands Inanna to bow low.

Can we dare to be more demanding?

I feel sacred rage emerging from the depths in the many social and political movements that are saying "no" to the domination and inequality that has been at play for so long. The Black Lives Matter Movement, the #MeToo movement, the horror and opposition to the oppression of women and girls in Afghanistan, the rage against the reversal of Roe v. Wade, which has overturned women's right to abortion in the USA. We are rising, we are becoming fierce and unsettling – we will not be held in the underworld anymore.

Chapter 10
HANGING ON THE HOOK

In birth, this is the place that midwives recognise as 'transition': where we think we cannot go on right before the baby arrives. When I gave birth to my first daughter, I remember looking up at the midwife and saying *"I can't do this"*. It was in that moment of *I can't,* that I submitted to the overwhelming power of birth. It felt like a birth quake, such a force of downward energy sweeping through my body. Looking back, of course it felt impossible, because what moves in birth is beyond us and part of us at the same time. We cannot 'do' birth: birth is something that takes us. This requires submission to the unknown, in a way that little else besides death does.

In the heroine's journey, sometimes we get stuck in this transition between death and rebirth for many years. If Ereshkigal doesn't get the empathy she needs, she will not grant the waters of life required for Inanna to rise and we can get caught on the hook unable to fully emerge into the light. Returning to Fiza Noor's story, she described this as being held in purgatory. We might get held in purgatory by a situation beyond our control, such as being a refugee waiting to be granted permission to stay, or living in a war zone. Or we can play a part in holding ourselves in purgatory for example, by staying in addictive cycles and not seeking help, or staying in abusive relationships. When we are dissociated we feel our body less, so it is more likely that we will override our needs and not always notice the pain we feel. As Fiza Noor articulates,

"I became a workaholic, I worked as much as possible. I made friends, but I had spent half my life in a disassociated space, in purgatory, and it was hard for me to truly connect to people. There are a lot of people who would call me a friend, who are like acquaintances to me, because the stage in my life when I met them I was not able to feel, because my body, myself, my mind has always been in disconnect, in a state of dissociation to protect myself. It's always been to protect myself and it's been since childhood."

Like Fiza, we can be quite high functioning on the outside and still be held captive in old trauma patterns, unable to thrive and move beyond the scratch in our record. We may seem to be doing fine, but inside part of us is trapped in the underworld. Particularly if we have experienced trauma or abuse in childhood, this state of freeze or dissociation may be 'normal' to us, it might be all we have ever known. With intergenerational trauma, the nervous system patterns that shape our lives can repeat themselves in all sorts of subtle and not so subtle ways. We can be held captive in the underworld for many years, never realising that there is another possibility.

I spoke to Tamara Albanna, who is from Iraq and has written about and worked with the Inanna-Ereshkigal myth extensively, she told me,

"I feel like perhaps this (being stuck in the underworld) is a cultural thing for us, that it's a martyrdom complex, especially with women. We carry so much stuff and we hold so much together, with family and everything. I have seen it with women in my family, especially where there is so much sacrificing going on. And Inanna was sacrificed, but she was resurrected. So where is our resurrection?... I feel like sometimes women don't seem to want to find compassion for themselves, because it's somehow seen as selfish. This is something I see in my own culture all the time, that everyone is put before them (women) and when everyone else is satiated and has everything they need, then they might look after themselves. But by then they're absolutely exhausted. It's a pattern that repeats. I think it's something we really need to look at more and talk about more and ask, why is that? And why do we need to drain our battery all the time before we look after ourselves?"

Tragically, patriarchy has come to thrive on women being kept down in the underworld. It is painfully ironic to me, that the country from which this powerful myth was birthed is actually a country whose women have been repeatedly sacrificed and are still massively oppressed.

Tamara's family had to flee Iraq in the 1990s, when she was only two years old. She spoke about the importance of keeping the Inanna story alive and the resilience of the Iraqi women,

"A lot of women seem to be in the underworld space, I feel like it's kind of a collective issue. Unfortunately, we are not always told the stories – especially Iraqis living in the diaspora – these really important stories about the Goddess, and that there even was a triple goddess in Arabia prior to the advent of Islam.

I heard about Inanna during my Masters studies. I was gathering statistics on violence against women and girls. I was doing a comparison between pre-war and post-war Iraq, and just after post-war was where I was focusing my studies. The Islamic state hadn't even started their genocidal rage at that point yet, and even then what I was seeing was quite bad. Several times, I broke down in my professor's office because of everything we had to read and listen to. And I was thinking, 'My goodness, there has to be more than this'.

I always refer to this CNN report by Arwa Damon, about when Al Qaeda had ravaged a city and there were only women and girls left. Arwa Damon managed to get into the city and she sat down with a family, and they told her basically that it was a systematic rape of the women and girls and the killing of all the men. So what they were trying to do was breed a new generation of fighters. And I'm listening to this and I just, I don't know, it started something, something clicked. I couldn't stop crying first of all, it was so devastating, then I was on this mission to find out more. I just kept diving deeper. I was contacting the military, contacting government at the highest levels with my professor. We were obsessed, wanting to know what the hell was happening to the women and girls there. And everywhere we went, we weren't able to get any information. And I am thinking: 'Are their lives really not worth it?' Had it not been for Arwa Damon's news report no one would know what happened to these women and girls, they would just be forgotten, again.

Somehow, I still don't know how, I ended up looking at the myth of Inanna again. I knew of Inanna, but I didn't have a deep dive, you know, it was very academically focused for me until that point. But I guess the timing was right. I re-read the myth again and sat with it for a while and I thought, 'Wow, how long have Iraq's women been going through the underworld? How long have they been sacrificed repeatedly, over and over again by various forces? Not just by their own, but outside forces and it continues and continues.'

The resilience of the Iraqi woman is unlike anything that I have ever seen – truly. It shocks me and it humbles me. It's like somehow, this grace in such chaos and such uncertainty, I feel like that's the Goddess running through it all. And that's how I observe it, because I think what else could it be? To have such strength and such courage to keep moving forward. Knowing that things are really dire, but somehow they still get up every day and go about their lives. That, for me, is a continuous source of inspiration."

I want to remember the Iraqi women who have been raped and forgotten. Women in other parts of the world who experience oppression and abuse beyond what I have ever had to endure. I feel this myth is an invitation to remember, reclaim and reconnect with the lost and forgotten parts of ourselves *and* the macrocosm of our humanity.

Remembering with empathy is the way we get off the hook.

Many people, like Inanna, do get released and flow back into life, even after the most shocking and traumatic underworld journeys. But some don't. I was really moved by Tamara's account of her mother's life.

"Intergenerational trauma is a big one. My mother has a lot of trauma, and that has caused our relationship to not be a very good one. We literally had to flee Iraq, it was quite traumatic. My father had to go first. My mother and I followed in a car through the desert. They told my father, 'They might not show up, they might get arrested, we don't know, we can't promise anything'. So I basically started my life with turmoil, in the diaspora, and being ripped away from my motherland. I was less than two years old. To this day, I don't understand why I have such a deep connection [to Iraq], as if I spent my whole life there, but I do. When we had to leave, my mother was young, all she knew was that she had to meet the man that she loved on the other side and get there, with her child in one piece. She said she just kept looking at the man that was driving and praying that he was a decent man and that we were going to make it on time. She said, 'It was hours and hours and I didn't sleep and I just held you really tight because I was terrified that something was going to happen'. And I knew, when she said those words, that there is such a deep trauma there.

So my mum left and she never went back: she has not seen her family for decades. When she left, she didn't know that it would be the last time. I know that this is huge, this is heavy for her...She told me that I cried a lot on that journey and she said, 'You were the one who was crying, because I couldn't cry, I had to keep myself composed. But it's like you were crying my tears as we were leaving.' She didn't know what was happening until she got to the other side when she was told there is no return for us, because bad things will happen.

They were forced into this new life, with no one and complete confusion, and they were very young, in their twenties. But, as difficult as my childhood was and all the trauma, and all the things that happened, I have deep empathy as well for all that they endured. And I know that if things could be different, things would be different, let's just say that. So it's just the way things went. And I had to accept that. It's taken a very long time. I have had to do the therapy and a lot of inner work in order to find relative peace. But it saddens me to think that my mother is still in some kind of turmoil. My mother lives in the underworld, that's what it feels like to me. She's just sort of taken up residence there. It's tragic really. But we all need to live our experiences, I can't do anything to help her out of that, she has to move through it. The only way I can possibly help anyone move through things, is by moving myself and doing the best that I can."

When we cannot, or do not, process our trauma we can spend a lifetime in the underworld. As Tamara names, it can be so difficult to witness someone we love trapped there and know that there is nothing we can do to help, unless and until they want to be helped. Sometimes it can become more comfortable to stay with what we know, rather than risk coming back to life. Life can feel very dangerous after being held on the hook for so long, because at least on the hook we know where we are. Or we forget what being truly alive feels like and get lost in despair and hopelessness. Or we lose our minds and land in dementia or psychosis.

I feel the Inanna-Ereshkigal myth offers a map that can encourage us to dare to live again, to dare to remember. One of the reasons I am so passionate about it, is that it does have an ascent. The second part of Inanna's journey teaches us that we can be released, that we can be resurrected, rise and thrive again. I feel it is of paramount importance that we remember that. As Tamara illuminates,

"I think of Inanna and Ereshkigal as two sides of the same person: it's looking in the mirror. When we descend, we are Ereshkigal, when we ascend we are Inanna. We need all aspects for balance. It's not possible to be in the light all the time and it's not healthy to be in the dark all the time either. And Inanna knew she was going to be sacrificed, she had to go to the deepest darkest depths. Parts of her had to die. Not saying that those aspects will no longer be a part of her, because they don't ever leave you, but she sort of became something else. She became stronger. And I really do believe it was a willing death, it was a necessary part of her story. Sometimes we have to go through hardships and owning that and having agency is so important. Even if it's something you don't want to have to deal with, when we say, 'Yes, I will deal with this, and I am going to learn from it and get through it', it is more empowering. Certainly Inanna is not a damsel in distress, or a figure who can be told what to do – at all. I wouldn't try it. For me, I feel like the Iraqi woman embodies that as well. Even with all that she has been through – don't mess with her."

I feel that what Tamara highlights so well here is that it is not the catalyst or the content of the descent that makes us a heroine, it's the way we *choose* to meet it, move towards it and find the courage to rise again.

Letting Ourselves Off the Hook

The number of times that I sit in the therapy room with people who say, *"this is not living"* or *"I can't carry on like this"*, while feeling desperately afraid of letting themselves off the hook. The cost being that we can knowingly or unknowingly become stuck in freeze, unable to leave the underworld. Toxic relationships, the wrong job, place, a story, unprocessed trauma, all these things can keep us hanging on the hook. For a while this survival strategy may be necessary, but in the long-term living in purgatory is one of the worst sorts of pain there is.

In terms of trauma, this can be perpetuated by minimising our experiences. Often people will say sentences that begin with, *"It was only..."* or *"It wasn't even that bad..."* or *"It sounds silly because..."*. This is a classic protection mechanism that can provide a necessary barrier to the wholeness of our experience for a while. But in the ascent, minimising can actually hold us back from truly thriving. In turn, this prevents us being receptive to the empathy that we need to flow forwards. As the myth teaches, empathy is the key to new life and empathy is not mind-led, it is a felt experience, one that can bring us home to our body. I think this is why, after Ereshkigal stakes Inanna, that she begins to make birthing sounds and names her pain, *"Oh my heart, oh my thighs, oh my belly!"* she cries. In the process of returning to her body, she feels all the aches and sensations that have been deadened for so long. In the spirit of our times, we often fail to see when a birth is taking place.

Actually, when people feel they are 'failing' they are often birthing.

We might believe that whilst we were battling on, surviving and keeping life going that we were 'doing fine' – but without the end to this façade how can we be transformed?

Our losses, mistakes and breakdowns carry so much shame or connotations of failure, which can actually stifle the process needed to integrate the experience. We might say, *"I thought I would be over this by now"*. But what we do not see is that we have entered the deep time of transformation, which moves slower than upperworld life. In our modern, secular world, we have largely lost the rituals and ceremony that mark these rites of passage, and with that, we have lost the markers, recognition and importance of our heroine's journeys. Books, stories and myths hold the power to rekindle that connection. As Tamara elucidates,

"The thing is with Inanna, I am thrilled when I see anyone talk and bring her name to their lips – for me it is an act of devotion. I think it's wonderful and I think that the world is hungry for it. And in particular, of course, the Western world is hungry for this because they had to emerge from Judeo-Christian thought and are still emerging from it. And look, in the US it's not a pretty picture: the constant degrading of women's rights and I am thinking, 'What is going on? What year are we living in?' I want people to continue to talk about Inanna. I want people to tell the story and look at how it applies to their own lives and, in that way, I hope it will continue going on and on through generations. That's my hope, at least, that the story never dies and that her name will always be spoken."

Chapter 11

MEETING ENKI – CONSCIOUSNESS AND THE IMPORTANCE OF THE MALE ALLY AND WITNESS

A story is 'holy,' and it is used as medicine. The story is not told to lift you up, to make you feel better, or to entertain you, although all those things can be true. The story is meant to take the spirit into a descent to find something that is lost or missing and to bring it back to consciousness again.

Clarissa Pinkola Estés, *Women Who Run with the Wolves*

The shadow side of any emotion is the place where we can become consumed by that emotion and get lost inside of it. I think this is one of the fears of the Dark Goddess: that she will devour us completely. In human terms, being devoured by something, be that drug addiction, psychosis, dementia, or deep depression, is frightening and for good reason: if we lose consciousness we can become stuck in the underworld.

Devouring energy is rife in modern times. Our human consumption and disregard for the laws of nature, that the Gatekeeper tells us very clearly *must not be questioned* is tipping us into our own collective destruction. There are many cautionary tales that warn of the cost of having too much. The story of the Hindu goddess Kali, who can be seen as another form of Ereshkigal, speaks to this.

The Story of Kali and Shiva

I first heard this myth told by Chameli Gad Ardagh in her TED Talk on "The Fierce Face of the Feminine". Shiva is presence and he uses his creativity and vulnerability to awaken Kali.

The story begins in the time of a great war between the gods and goddesses and some powerful demons. The demons were so powerful that if they were cut and a drop of their blood fell to the earth, more demons would sprout. The goddesses were almost defeated when Durga realised that she needed to birth an even more fierce aspect of the feminine. And so, from her third eye, she birthed Kali. Kali is the Hindu triple goddess of birth, preservation and destruction. She holds seemingly opposite polarities within her. Kali enters the battle, killing the demons and using her long tongue to lick up the blood before more demons can sprout. But, as she tastes the blood, she becomes intoxicated and cannot stop killing: she becomes lost in a frenzy.

Durga calls on Shiva, who is married to Kali, and implores him to stop her. He tries to distract her, to tame her, to appeal to her consciousness, but nothing works. He feels defeated. In a last attempt to reach her, he lies down on the ground in front of her and reveals his soft belly. Just as Kali is about to stamp on him, she stops. She wakes up. This act of submission and vulnerability of the masculine awakens her back to herself and the world is saved.

Kali without Shiva is destruction; Kali with Shiva is medicine.

Chameli Gad Ardagh

Meeting Enki

In the Inanna-Ereshkigal myth, Enki is similar to Shiva. He acts as a male witness and ally to the feminine. He is the creative, empathic masculine who immediately shares Ninshubur's concern for Inanna and wants to help. As Sylvia Brinton Perera names,

There is one 'father' in the Descent myth who is helpful: Enki. His name means 'lord of the earth' (like Poseidon) [...] He lives deep in the abyss. He is a remarkable divinity. In Sumer, his waters were equated with the

engendering power of semen and amniotic fluid [...] Enki is the generative, creative, playful, empathetic male.

In opposition to the Sky Gods, Enki feels grieved by his daughter's plight in the underworld. He is the male that has been initiated into the masculine and feminine aspects of his own being. He has entered the depths and flow of his own waters and he embodies emotional grace.

"From under his fingernail Father Enki brought forth dirt.

He fashioned the dirt into a kugarra, a creature neither male or female form.

From under the fingernail of his other hand he brought forth dirt.

He fashioned the dirt into a galatur, a creature neither male or female form."

These creatures, these emissaries from God, are sexless. Diane Wolkstein suggests that this is so that they do not flout the infertility laws of the underworld which means that they can pass the gates of the *kur* on behalf of Enki. In terms of boundaries, I feel it is significant that he sends emissaries, that Enki doesn't go and rescue Inanna himself – because it's not about him. Rather, it's about his creativity, and in honouring that, he does not interfere with the heroine's individuation process. He can stand beside her as an ally, but cannot rescue her and nor does he try. He does not enmesh himself in her process, or rob her of her sovereignty in any way. He has integrity and he honours the boundaries of the underworld. He cannot, and should not, trespass there (unless he is being initiated himself). Only his emissaries can enter. In terms of therapy this is key. If a therapist becomes too involved (or sexually involved) with a client when they are in the fragile depths of initiation, they rob them of the individuation process and prevent the heroine completing her ascent.

Enki instructs the *galatur* and *kugarra* to empathise with Ereshkigal who he says will be making birthing sounds. They are told to provide a mirror for Ereshkigal's labour pains (metaphorical or physical). This is absolutely crucial. An empathic witness can make the difference between us getting stuck in the underworld or the waters of new life being released.

Yoga practice can teach us how to embody the *kugarra* and *galatur* in ourselves. As Angela Farmer described to me,

> "My practice now is simply to meet, one at a time, the painful places
> in my body and see if, instead of forcing or judging, as was the old
> pattern, I can soften, feel and listen until they unwind and release.

The *kugarra* and *galatur*, are the parts of me that empathise with that place. Once seen and heard, it intuitively finds its own way back to the light. Our busy and controlling front brain, kind of 'dissolves down' into the body and, like a flashlight, guides us to what needs attention. I love the way that these two tiny creatures sit next to Ereshkigal and do nothing but just listen, giving her full respect by simply repeating what she says."

This deep listening is incredibly medicinal for Ereshkigal and in gratitude, she offers them a gift of the water of life. This represents shakti, or *jouissance*, the feminine flow of energy, the river of our lives which can flow again. This is a fundamental teaching of the myth: only by allowing death can we enter new life.

Enki has dirt under his fingernails, he is a gardener, he is not afraid to put his hands in the Earth. His playfulness has an innocence that we often associate with children, but actually, we all hold innocence whatever our age. I don't believe that innocence is something we can outgrow. It is the energy inside us that is not tarnished by difficult life experiences. It is the reason my Nannan, now one hundred years old, still talks about "old people" as if they are other than her. It is a shame that we have a tendency to only associate innocence with children, or those who are a bit naïve. Actually, the root of the word innocence means *no-harm*. For me, innocence is the part of us that is inherently non-harming to others, but also the place within us that is not touched by the suffering that happens to us in life. Even if we have suffered severe trauma and abuse, there is the potential to contact the part of ourselves that is still innocent. Despite whatever horrific things might have happened, there is an enduring innocence that remains untouched. I believe Enki symbolises the part of us that knows this.

Enki is also vital as a male ally for a woman in crisis. As a woman, I needed a male witness who was not afraid of my transformation, and I believe that this has to come from outside our family system. As we descend, the old formative patterns being unearthed often put a strain on our personal relationships. All parents and caregivers are human and have blind spots. As we mature, we need elders who can be a guide for the parts of us that our parents couldn't see or meet. I think it's essential that we have elders that are not kin, because anyone closely related to us has, as Stephen Jenkinson puts it, "too much skin in the game". An elder needs a healthy separation from us, if they are going to be a true guide in our life.

I found Enki in the form of a male psychotherapist and Hakomi practitioner, John Hillman, who was my ally and compassionate witness in the depths. When we sit beside someone immersed in the underworld, some part of us touches that place with them. It may evoke our own memories, vulnerability, emotions and wounds. Any therapist knows that the material our clients bring to us can bring up our own stuff, this is a natural part of the process and why supervision is so essential.

In some therapeutic modalities there can be a tendency for the therapist to occupy the role of expert, or Sky God. I feel Enki is the antithesis of this. He offers partnership with, not domination over, Inanna. He is an ally and a beholder. Not a superior, but a trusted companion who has himself been initiated. My therapist held within his beingness a sense of deep acceptance and a reverence for all that we do not know. This transmission was communicated in words and through the creative use of poetry, but also beyond words. In short, what he brought was embodied loving presence. Having an external male witness was an essential aspect of my heroine's journey that helped me form a different relationship with the masculine on the outer and inner. This has also had a significant impact on how I now relate to structure, containment and self-holding.

I would suggest that male beholders and allies are essential for our collective transformation. This kind of work is so sparsely populated with males, which is a great loss. The myth teaches us that it is totally possible and necessary for females to initiate and behold other females, and that women hold both yin and yang energy. But I do not think that this makes male witnesses obsolete. Far from it, we are one humanity, and, personally, I need male allies, male presence and brothers to stand beside me.

I am heartened by Enki's creativity, emotionality and playfulness which models a different kind of masculine than the hero of our popularised patriarchal tales. As ecological storyteller and author, Sophie Strand explores,

For too long masculinity has been conflated with patriarchy. Over the years as I researched [...] I realized there was a rich history of mythology, folklore, and fairy tales that suggested that prior to patriarchy and imperialism there had been a biodiversity of masculinities deeply tied to vegetal wisdom, fermentation, multi-species collaboration, lunar cycles, and ecstatic festivity. Long before the sword-wielding heroes of legend readily cut down forests, slaughtered the old deities, and vanquished their enemies, there were playful gods, animal-headed kings, mischievous lovers, trickster harpists, and shape shifting magicians with flowering wands. Like underground mycelial systems, these wilder, more magical modes of the masculine have always been threaded through the underworld, waiting to fruit up when the time is opportune.

What would a more biodiverse landscape of masculinity mean for our evolution as a species? Sophie Strand's imagery offers a revitalising alternative to the monoculture of the strong masculine. I hear from the men I know and work with that they too are craving new narratives of masculinity and are discovering and creating them from inside their own bodies and relationships. I love the image of the masculine *fruiting up* out of the Earth and the underworld, not down from the sky. This, like Enki, signifies the potential for an Earth-bound, Earth-loving, rewilding of the masculine which is so needed.

We need men. We need men as the dominant people in our patriarchal culture to ally those of us who are not male. We need men to see that misogyny is not only a women's issue. We need men to take responsibility for making spaces more inclusive and safe for women. We need men to interrupt their fellow men when they see ignorance or hear harmful derogatory language being spoken. To protect those who are physically less strong than them, and to become more intimate with their sexual energy and shadow, so that they can become allies.

Our Sky God culture has meant that many men are emotionally wounded. When I have witnessed men in the descent, they often use metaphors of sinking ships and sea themes. I believe this is symbolic of how vast and consuming it can feel to men re-entering the depths of their root chakras and their emotional underworld. Still to this day, to be more male is to be elevated and to be female is to be denigrated, meaning that to survive and be a success, both men and women still default to rejecting what we perceive as more feminine traits and expression. At puberty, or even before, many boys send their emotional bodies underground and I believe that this thwarts their empathy towards self and others. The danger being that when we are emotionally disconnected, we can harm others or know that others are being harmed without fully feeling it.

If we can't bear to feel, we have to dominate.

Enki represents an important aspect of our humanity: he is the awakened empathic inner and outer masculine that can act in the world in compassionate action. He can play, he knows his own magic, he can ride the waves of emotion and he can behold the feminine. We need his presence, vulnerability and creativity. We need awakened, initiated males who are ready to imaginatively embody a different way.

To become an Enki, a man must himself descend to be initiated by Ereshkigal. Like Inanna, he must shed old identities, submit to the fullness of all his feelings, grieve the hurts he has caused to himself and others, and awaken to his shadow. This is symbolised later in the ascent, when Inanna sacrifices her husband Dumuzi, and sends him to the underworld (see Chapter Thirteen). It is not enough for the feminine to be initiated alone.

Journalling enquiry: Meeting Enki

How is Enki present in your life?

What is your relationship with your creativity?

What is a creative edge for you right now?

Do you have an external Enki who supports you? If not, would you like one?

What do you feel about the possibility of being beheld by a man?

Anything else that has come up for you in this enquiry?

RISING – THE ASCENT

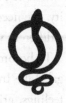

It's not so much the solstice
as the morning after
when light comes after the longest night
and the clock is not what you think it should be
and you could not remain asleep with your mind
spinning in the darkness that comes
after difficult days
when nothing is what you thought or wanted
and the thing you wish would let go
will not.
There are lessons in endurance,
but what are they?
In the tunnel, you can't see,
except for the step that waits
in front of you. The only thing to do.
Wake and step forward into this morning's darkness
without certainty or security, with only what you have
in this moment. There may be no other.
Whatever comes next will be what is.
And this darkness is turning even in this
long still moment as you watch
the sun being reborn.

"Turning" by MJ Adams

Chapter 12

REBIRTH, EMERGENCE AND BECOMING A VIRGIN

The rivers of life have started to flow, which initiates Inanna's rebirth. But, as we have seen, Ereshkigal is a teacher of boundaries, and as Inanna emerges from the underworld she is flanked by the *galla* demons whose job it is to ensure that Inanna sends another to the underworld to take her place. Like Enki's *kugarra* and *galatur*, the *galla* are also neither male nor female. The *galla* are devouring demons, and they want to be fed. They carry the part that exists in all humans, that wants what we want, no matter what the cost. They hold the energy of the destroyer part of Kali untempered by Shiva, they are the devouring aspect of Ereshkigal without empathy, they are the part of animals that will savage another animal for survival. They are indiscriminate about their hunger. They cannot be bribed, bargained with, extinguished or escaped from. They exist to enforce the laws of the underworld and they stay until it is done.

Like the unequivocal energy of the descent, these *galla* hold in place the unequivocal sacrifice of the ascent. They are enduring, and if we do not abide by the transformative energy as it moves us, we literally become *haunted by our demons*. There are many ways this can play out in our lives, it could show up as bitterness and resentment, or the insatiable pursuit of revenge on those who we feel have done us wrong. It could be the abyss of grief that consumes us and possibly leads us to take our own life, or a relapse into destructive addictions.

If we do not make a sacrifice, we may have to become the sacrifice.

In this part of the journey we are acutely vulnerable, and if we do not get the help and support we need, it is very easy to fall foul to the energy of demons, be that in the destruction of ourselves and/or others. But, if we bring our consciousness to this emergence, the *galla* can be a call towards growth. They dictate that we cannot emerge the same as we were before, we have to relinquish whatever is not in service of the journey. They demand a price and the price will be paid.

Being faced with this just as we emerge can be exhausting. Having lost so much in the descent we are already fatigued. To discover that more sacrifices need to be made is daunting to say the least. Many women who shared their stories with me named how lengthy this process of sacrifice and emergence can be. The concentric cycles within the greater cycle are considerable, as we pendulate back and forth between what we were, and how we used to do things, and what we are becoming and how we are learning to do things differently.

Pendulation is an important part of trauma work. Learning to move between opposites, and find a way out of the stuckness, is the way we unfreeze what has become frozen within us. Peter Levine describes pendulation as the movement between contraction and expansion. As we emerge there will be moments when we open up to life again, but then we will likely retract back inwards again. Moving between polarities is an organic way to gradually process and become more aware of what is moving in us. Learning to pendulate between known patterns (even 'unhealthy' ones) and stretching into new frontiers of ourselves is important. If we rush our sacrifices we can end up sending key parts of ourselves to the underworld again. But if we are patient, slowly, we can begin to integrate what we have learned from our descent in a way that is digestible and not obliterating to our self. As Claire Patrick, described:

"It's been a five-year sacrifice, because I had to let go of the version of myself and what kind of life I thought I would have, in terms of career. Being very achievement- and career-driven and hard work-focused was how I was. Over the last five years I keep trying: I go through phases where I release my work for a period and then I get drawn back in, and I release it for a period and I get drawn back in. So it's still a question, on the one hand I am here to tell stories, but the world I have to occupy to do that is hard to navigate. So I am still integrating it and it's five years on."

Boundaries and Sacrifice

Emerging is also a process of discovering what needs to be protected and what needs to be sacrificed into order to live more and more authentically. The *galla* that flank us as we emerge from the underworld provoke us to step into our authority and invoke new boundaries. However, the need to earn money and belong are strong and genuine needs that sometimes conflict with our newly emerging self. As we rise, we endeavour to find a way to embody the lessons that we are still in the process of integrating *and* be in the upperworld at the same time.

It can be a struggle, because the world has not changed, but we have.

In this phase, we are in many ways like a newborn. There is a fragility and necessary flailing. I often compare this part of the ascent to the springtime of the menstrual cycle, the first few days after our bleed. At this point, we might feel energised and inspired, but if we run with this energy too quickly, it can leave us feeling vulnerable and overly exposed. If the first shoots of spring rise too soon, a frost can kill them. This is a microcosm of the kind of vulnerability we feel as we start to emerge from the underworld. We feel our sap rising, but we are still young in our new form. And yet, paradoxically, a part of us has matured and been seasoned in a way that only the underworld can flavour a human.

When a woman returns from the underworld journey, when she has witnessed the pain and indiscriminate fury of her dark sister, and suffered her own dismemberment and death, she does not return with all-loving sweetness and radiant light. Around her cling Ereshkigal's demons, emissaries of the dark; we see them in the deepened furrows on her brow, the tension she holds in her body, her darkened eyes, and cheeks scored by tears. These are the marks she bears as she returns; this is the woman who must search for a sacrifice, and she will not be released by the clinging demons until she finds one.

Linda Hartley, *Servants of the Sacred Dream*

The Virgin

When we flower again into the ascent, we are virgins. In her book *The Moon and the Virgin*, Nor Hall tells us that the Latin and Greek etymologies refer to a virgin as a woman not belonging to any man, but to herself. She who is true to her own nature and instinct. This is what Inanna has become and is becoming.

A virgin is a woman, one in herself, owned by no man, author of her own life, creatress of her own destiny

Marija Gimbutas, *The Civilisation of the Goddess*

She is not dependent on the reactions of others to define her own being. The virginal woman is not just a counterpart to the male, whether father, lover or husband. She stands as an equal in her own right.

Nancy Qualls-Corbett, *The Sacred Prostitute: Eternal Aspect of the Feminine*

Inanna embodies her virginity as she emerges from the underworld, not because she is young, untouched or naïve, but because she has been initiated by her own dark material into her own wholeness. This is a turnaround of everything that patriarchal narratives have imposed onto the term virgin. In modern culture, a woman is usually considered to be a virgin until she has had penetrative sex with a man. Again, man initiating woman into her sexuality. In the USA and other places, it is still perfectly legal to have 'hymen checks' carried out by Sky God medical professionals who can apparently deem whether a woman is 'chaste' or not. Of course, it's all rubbish, because the hymen can break from exercise, using a tampon or, god forbid, self-pleasuring. But still, our society tries to perpetuate the ownership of women's bodies and sexuality through these kinds of false and oppressive narratives.

The heroine is one who has remembered, reclaimed and reconnected with her unfettered red thread. She has been initiated into the spirit of the depths by her dark sister, and walks with newfound, embodied authority into the upperworld. This rearrangement of self goes way beyond the mind, it reverberates in our cells, our breath, our heartbeat, in matter or *mater* (meaning mother).

The heroine is learning and asserting new boundaries, feeling and allowing all her feelings, and using her voice to define her new ground. This is a rebirth in the most visceral way: our nervous system, our responses, our sexuality, our voice, our relationships have changed, and are changing. It does not mean we are perfect, on the contrary we are awake to our human flaws, perhaps more acutely than ever. But we have touched something inside ourselves, a knowing so deep it can hardly be articulated. It is beyond words, beyond 'knowing', an inward state that has nothing and everything to do with physical beingness. It is what the Catholic mystic Thomas Merton called the *pointe verge*, which is the hiding place of God/Goddess within us. It is a place inside us that cannot be shared directly by anyone else and that we cannot pin down, but that we can catch glimpses of from within. Once we have touched this place, we are changed irreversibly by it. It is a moment of grace and grace just comes, it does not knock – it arrives. Spontaneously. And then, is gone again, but it leaves a lasting impression.

> *If I never see it again – nor ever feel it*
> *I know that it is –*
> *and that if once it hailed me, it ever does,*
> *And so it is myself I want to turn in that direction*
> *Not as in towards a place, but it was a tilting inside myself*
> *as one turns a mirror to flash the light to where it isn't –*
> *I was blinded like that – and swam in what shone at me*
> *Only able to endure it by being no one*
> *And so specifically myself I thought I'd*
> *die from being loved like that.*

"Annunciation" by Marie Howe

Through my descent I encountered this place inside myself. It is the *"serene lake inside myself"* that Claire Patrick referred to in her story. And I believe that Inanna has experienced this, she has surrendered to it and she emerges a virgin, in the truest sense of the word.

Like the virgin forest, she is full of her own life force, full of potential, and pregnant.

Marion Woodman, *The Pregnant Virgin*

Pregnant, not necessarily with a baby, though in Sophie Jane Hardy's case she was, but pregnant meaning full of herself, pregnant with her own creative potential. Therefore, virginity is not something that can be given or taken away: it is who we are.

For me, this phase of the ascent was a whole combination of things. I emerged with a stronger devotion than ever before, utter determination and a calling to support others to reconnect to their feminine ground of being. But this was also combined with sorrow, and an equally strong sense of vulnerability; a not knowing how my life, my work and myself, now looked in the world. I felt like a new, lesser-known shape that was me, but in the absence of so much that I used to call "me" there was a weird freedom and also strangeness in my body and way of being. I felt more sturdy and robust, but also, embryonic and impossibly fresh to the world. Ereshkigal has given us the harshest lessons and we are fortified by her raw clarity, which we must now refine into conscious action as we rise.

Chapter 13

MEETING DUMUZI – THE SACRIFICE OF THE ARROGANT MASCULINE

Our rising holds uncanny echoes of the descent and at times we may feel like we are going backwards. There are so many cycles within the wider cycle, so many opportunities to more deeply imprint and embody what we have learnt and are learning. It's non-linear and sometimes we might feel like we are all over the place – support is key. To illustrate this, throughout the next two chapters I highlight the moments that I feel correspond with the gates of the underworld and how they might show up as we rise.

As Inanna emerges, the first person she encounters is Ninshubur, her loyal witness, who has been in anguish over her loss. Ninshubur has been utterly committed to Inanna, so when the *galla* demons try to take her, the decision is clear. Inanna says no.

The voices we remembered in Gate Three support our rising. Asserting our no is a powerful part of the ascent. Through the no, we can better protect ourselves and stand firm in what we need, which is an essential part of rising in our integrity.

Then Inanna encounters her sons. They too have grieved the loss of their mother. I feel Inanna's sons represent the part of our inner masculine that can be reverent towards the feminine. Inanna will not allow them to be sacrificed either.

Finally, she arrives at Dumuzi, her husband, who is sitting on Inanna's throne. In complete contrast to Ninshubur and her sons, Dumuzi has not visibly grieved the loss of his wife. Instead he has happily usurped Inanna and shows no humility or sorrow. Therefore, he is the one she must sacrifice.

Sacrificing Dumuzi can be the most challenging part of rising. The descent has changed Inanna's relationship with the feminine. She is no longer dominating and exiling Ereshkigal, she is including her and is even beginning to be guided by her presence. Now her relationship with the masculine needs to change so that the divergent parts of her can come into a supportive relationship.

It is thought this myth was written as Sumerian society transitioned from being a matrilineal society to a patriarchy. It is interesting to me that Ninshubur goes to the Sky Gods for help: female elders do not feature in the myth. Some writers suggest that this was Enheduanna's observation about the changing power-er structures in society. And now Dumuzi, Inanna's husband, is sitting on *her* throne. Symbolically, could this point to the ways that males and the masculine were taking over space that the feminine and females had previously shared?

> *In patriarchal culture, Dumuzi's prominence on that*
> *throne and the idea that he has the right to it has been so*
> *commonplace, for so long, that culturally, we believe it.*

At this point we are able to take responsibility for our own parts. It was we who rejected and blamed Ereshkigal, we who elevated and colluded with the Sky Gods. It is unsurprising then that we might go on to repeat this pattern internal-ly, and with our lovers. The sacrifice of Dumuzi is the process of discovering how this is true for us. That is not to negate the very real impact of women's cultural and historical oppression, but as we rise we hold awareness of this, alongside our ability to see how we have helped perpetuate it – so that we can be instrumental in the authorship of a new story.

Dumuzi is the masculine that will not surrender to his emotions and is es-tranged from the dark feminine. He is the one inside us who is well-versed in the world of patriarchy, who, to some degree, likes the order of things and does not want to engage with the underworld. He would rather stay safe above ground. He is the allure of putting up a front, being right, superior or avoiding change, and what's more, he will ignore what is in front of his face to do it.

Collectively, I see Dumuzi as the face of society that cannot look at its shadow and cannot, or will not, empathise with others. He is the politician who gives evasive answers rather than compassionate replies, he is the media who actively keeps the feminine split in two, he is the dictator that won't step down – he is the one who serves himself. Internally, he is our blind arrogance, the one inside us that believes we should be immune – to suffering, to ageing, to being like everyone else.

Recognising Dumuzi

For some women, recognising Dumuzi as an internal aspect of ourselves is more complex because we are so heavily conditioned to renounce our arrogance, to stay small, to stay safe – taking up the inferior or apologetic stance is a well-known position for women and girls. Whereas, in patriarchal society, males are generally encouraged from a young age to cultivate the visible Dumuzi, the elevated, confident, dominant, male leader. Even now, females are largely encouraged to follow, support, or be attracted to Dumuzi. Or conversely, protect against and reject him – but never be him. The cost being

if we are always in a dominator dynamic with some external form
of Dumuzi, it makes our inner Dumuzi very difficult to feel.

I can feel my resistance to naming this, I don't want to believe it is still true. But studies show how women and girls still tend to underestimate ourselves, whilst men and boys tend to overestimate themselves. And I see it in the women in my life, who still doubt themselves in ways that their male counterparts do not so readily. Thankfully, it is changing and there will always be exceptions to the rules. But for many women, Dumuzi will likely first appear as an external male, or woman with a prominent masculine energy, who we have pedestalled, been abused by, have been stuck under, are in love with, or are in some sort of toxic power dynamic with, that we have to sacrifice.

In the Sky Gods, the elevated masculine is easier to see, yet, in our personal lives, Dumuzi is likely to be someone or something that we feel resistant to sacrificing. Sadly, our oppressors are often closer to us than we think and the closer they are the harder they are to see – they are all too commonly people we know and love. This is Inanna's husband, she is wed to him. Though in our particular stories we may not be actually married to Dumuzi, we are emotionally attached to him. But being attached to him does not automatically mean that he is supportive to us. On the contrary, at this moment, Dumuzi's arrogance prevents him from working on our behalf. But the feelings we have for him are likely complex and multi-layered which can make it very difficult to extrapolate ourselves from the relationship.

Dumuzi energy is rife in our modern world. He is what we are encouraged to strive for: the individualistic, successful, unshakable masculine. To challenge his narrative is to stand for something visibly different, which is both exciting and can make rising in our feminine feel very exposing. In a sense, this is the way that Inanna's nakedness continues above ground. The descent wrenches the sleep from our eyes and, once opened, we cannot close to what we have seen. Whereas Dumuzi is cosseted by his own ignorance. He is the parts of our lives and relationships that we still have to address.

The sacrifice of Dumuzi is the next uncomfortable step that we have to take in our outer lives to actualise the transformations that have happened internally. As we face the king, there are echoes of Gate One. What crown does Dumuzi hold at this point in our journey that we still believe we need to hold on to, or aspire to?

Being Seen

Dumuzi may not be able to see us. But we now see him. Inanna sees him. She sees and can finally admit, his inability to see her. Like in Gate Two, something we could not previously see is now unveiled. The descent has awakened us to some of our patterns, habitual prejudices and ignorance, as we rise this contin-ues, calling us to take greater responsibility for our actions.

For many women, this seeing is in itself a privilege. We have to be in a place of reasonable physical and financial safety to be able to rise. If we are surviving and unsupported, it might not be possible. Many of us are in relationship with an arrogant or abusive other that is taking up more space than belongs to him. Be that at work, in an intimate relationship, in the family dynamic or in the wider world. He takes what is not his to elevate himself, by putting down others, taking land, roles or the monopolising of ideas and resources, and usually a com-bination of these. The key is: he excludes consciousness of Inanna, his partner and wife, to do it. He cannot, or will not, see her. But now Inanna sees him, it empowers and informs her next steps.

Once we begin to see our relationship with Dumuzi through new eyes, we have to feel the feelings we have about it. In the myth, Dumuzi has been Inanna's husband and lover: to be unseen by him in this way is significant. In the story of Kali and Shiva we saw the importance of the empathic masculine as the beholder of the feminine. Enki also demonstrates this. At this stage, Dumuzi is the opposite. To finally recognise the way he exists in our lives can be a deeply destabilising part of the journey, when, on a tough day, it is tempting to go back to our old, known ways of being. But to drift back into the old shape would be to abort the final part of the cycle.

Dumuzi shows no reverence for Inanna's journey and it is for this reason that she knows that he too must go to the underworld and bow to the laws that exist there.

I call this part of the ascent 'the second wave of grief'. The first waves were more internal and personal, they happened at the epicentre of who we are. When the second wave comes, the ripple effects move out even further and change the terrain of our upperworld life. Some of us will feel exalted by this, but it is usually intermingled with loss. We saw this in Jacinta's story (Gate Seven) when, even though she had conviction about her choice to sacrifice her family, culture and living in her village, she still felt grief and loss over it – a part of her even felt that she had betrayed them.

But if she hadn't sacrificed them, she would have had to sacrifice herself.

This is the decision Inanna is faced with.

Dumuzi is the part of us, or others, that does not value, or perhaps even have the capacity to recognise, feminine wisdom. But regardless of this, we now have to show up as we are. Similar to Gate Five, we must dare to do all the things we fear we can't, or shouldn't do. This means trusting ourselves to do *our* work and live *our* lives, *our* way. For me, this meant, resting more, doing less. It was being more assertive. It involved discovering, owning and voicing my sexual desires, and deepening intimacy with my husband. It was being visibly creative and offering my work out to others. It was charging adequately for my work. It was actualising the lessons of Gate Six, by being kinder to my body and following a more cyclical practice. And it was realising my connection to source – to magic.

This part of the journey asks us to find the faith to stand in our authority *alongside* our not knowing and vulnerability. Then, our inner masculine and feminine start to find a new dance and we are drawn to webs of connection with those who support us when we stumble.

When we sacrifice Dumuzi, we become more visible to ourselves and others. Any residual relationships with the masculine – inner or outer – that are holding us back, have to change or be sacrificed completely. When Inanna instructs the *galla* to take Dumuzi, she steps into her authority in a very visible way.

In the light of day, for all to see, she sacrifices the king.

Dancing with the inner masculine and feminine

This is a visualisation that I was first guided through by Jules Heavens. It helps us to uncover the masculine and feminine within, gain insight into how they are in relationship and uncover anything that may need to be seen or healed. It can include movement if you feel the impulse. To begin, find a comfortable place to settle into your body and close your eyes, or have them at half-mast.

You begin in a room, look around and acquaint yourself with the space. How do you feel as you enter it?

Then a woman enters the room, look at her, what does she look like, what is she wearing, how does she move? She begins dancing. Notice her movements, how do they feel, what do they evoke in you?

Then a man enters the room, look at him, what does he look like, what is he wearing, how does he move? He begins to dance. Notice his movements, how do they feel, what do they evoke in you?

As these two figures dance notice how they move. Are they together, or apart, what is the dynamic between them? What do you feel in your body? How are you breathing? Anything else that you notice?

Eventually, the dance ends and you come back into your space. Open your eyes and take time to emerge. Then spend some time journalling about what you experienced. How do your inner masculine and feminine currently dance within you?

Becoming More Resourced

Dumuzi is referred to as being a shepherd. In biblical stories and other fables, shepherds are leaders chosen by God. Sheep are defenceless creatures and this part of the masculine is the one who is supposed to look after the flock. But in modern Western patriarchal culture, he doesn't always honour this role because he is estranged from the feminine and without connection to her, he cannot be truly compassionate to himself or others.

This part of the ascent calls us to readdress how we are resourced and supported in life – that includes economic stability. Sheep were vital commodities in Sumerian civilisation, for wool, meat and trade. Dumuzi holds wealth. Money is often associated with the masculine in terms of the structure and support it provides to us. For most people, money is a key relationship in our lives that has a big impact on our freedom of choice and how resourced we feel. In *Fix the System, Not the Women,* author Laura Bates outlines how systemic oppression plays out in our society and the impact on women and girls,

Women are dramatically more likely than men to be underpaid (they make up two thirds of workers twenty-five and over who are paid less that the minimum wage), but they are much less likely than men to make an official complaint about it.

Sacrificing Dumuzi is the way we learn to make our complaints, look at our relationship with money and structure, ask for what we need and value ourselves more (even in the face of those who do not value us).

It is how we become more resourced.

Though there is an increasing number of wealthy, influential women in the modern world, the richest most powerful people in Western society are still predominantly men. Looking at the Inanna story in a modern capitalist context, having been disowned by the Sky Gods, Inanna may feel she has to hang onto Dumuzi, (however he shows up in our lives) as a way of maintaining her power and income. Dumuzi, as an actual person, job, place or role could represent the last thread of security in an upperworld culture dominated by men and masculine values. This is a fear – real or imagined – that we have to reckon with as we rise.

Understanding It's Not Personal

Dumuzi is part of the façade of the masculine, which has had to cut off from emotionality and empathy to survive. This could be part of the reason that he cannot acknowledge Inanna's descent: he only sees himself.

I have found that one of the most difficult things for clients who have suffered abuse, is to eventually face the reality that it wasn't about them. When we are abused, excluded, hurt, we tend to carry the story that it is because of something *we* did, something shameful about *us*. This narrative, though painful, still puts us at the centre of what happened. But actually, in that moment, the abuser doesn't see us. Just as Dumuzi doesn't see Inanna. He has lost – or is estranged from – the capacity to see beyond himself. To admit that we have been objectified by another, that all they could see was their need, their desire, that we were simply an object – dehumanised – is excruciating.

All humans need to know our internal Dumuzi, so that we can take responsibility for him – women included. But I feel that for men, this is an evolutionary edge that desperately needs bringing to light because too many women are being killed by men. Dumuzi says, *"It's not my responsibility, it's up to her to change her behaviour to fix it."* Both men and women have bought into this narrative. It needs to be sacrificed. How do men come closer to this part of themselves? How do women notice how we collude with it? These are questions that need to be asked. The #notallmen is Dumuzi at play in our modern world. Psychotherapist and author of, *The Devil You Know*, Gwen Adshead states,

When we hear about somebody who has killed a child, or done something else terrible, horrible or scary […] there is a very strong wish to push them away and not see them as human like us. Try and distance ourselves. 'I'm not like that, that couldn't be a person like me'. But that dehumanisation is actually, ironically, something that allows people to do cruel things to other people. So that dehumanisation process is something we have to be very careful about.

Ultimately, Dumuzi's charisma covers his weakness and fear. I have worked with many women whose male partners and/or male family members, like Dumuzi, cannot see – or at least cannot admit to seeing – the changes happening in the women they love. When these women, like Inanna, start to assert themselves, it is not uncommon for their male counterparts to either reject them or slip off into hiding. If Dumuzi cannot face Inanna, his next solution is to avoid her. He may deny the need to change, protest that it is her problem not his, or claim that everything is fine the way it is. Denial is strong in the elevated masculine.

Those of us who are highly empathic may find it difficult not to overcompensate for Dumuzi at this crucial moment. This is part of *our* arrogance because it is based on the superior position of thinking we *know* what is right for another. But how can we possibly know what he needs? We might feel like sacrificing him is abandoning him, which can feel unbearable. But he is a grown man: if he doesn't descend, he won't change. And if we don't sacrifice him, nor will we.

The sacrifice, then, is a key part of being responsible for our own change first, and facing the fact that not everyone will have the capacity, or desire, to meet us there.

Making the Sacrifice

Our power is the agreement to see and honour ourselves, which may not change the system or others overnight, but will certainly change us and how resourced we feel. Inanna is the bold feminine, who asserts herself and is learning to take care of her own needs. She is the one in us that understands that some risk is crucial for growth. Largely, we only discover we are safe once we have taken a risk. This is why the heroine's journey is so fortifying, because after shedding, grieving, facing our worst fears, and getting to know our patterns and bodies better, we discover a new level of safety within ourselves: a holding deeper than we have ever felt. But, like Gate Seven, this stage of our rising necessarily tests those roots.

Inanna has been to the underworld to reclaim what is in exile inside herself. And she was slain because of it. This time, *she* is not the one who will be sacrificed. Instead she must now make the sacrifice. This is a highly unusual place for women to stand. When she prepares to sacrifice Dumuzi, she steps out of being done to, and steps into being the do-er. She shifts from surrender to action and in doing so she is the protagonist of her own rising.

This is a radical moment for many women. A terrifyingly exhilarating moment. To sacrifice Dumuzi, she must be in her agency with unapologetic conviction.

For so long, I was not identified with being the one who takes space, the sacrificer, the authority. I was always the one rebelling, rejecting or being a victim/prey. To sacrifice Dumuzi was to write a new story. I became the author of what came next, and the author of this book. It's scary and thrilling territory. I spent so long waiting for permission, waiting to be seen. To make the sacrifice is to admit that,

no one will give us permission.

Sacrificing Dumuzi is a fundamental demonstration of the willingness to consolidate our power. It is the way in which we continue to build trust with our newly forming self, bringing our masculine and feminine into a new relational dynamic – a partnership.

Can we dare to make that final leap to freedom?

Chapter 14

EMBODYING THE SNAKE: RETURNING TO LIFE

If all symbols are really functions and signs of things imbued with energy, then the serpent is, by analogy, symbolic of energy itself – of force pure and simple; hence its ambivalence and multivalences.

Juan Cirlot, *A Dictionary of Symbols*

When Inanna changes the power dynamic, Dumuzi's front crumbles in the face of her clarity – his vulnerability is revealed. As the *galla* go to seize him, he turns into a snake and slithers off to hide. When the charisma falls, we get to meet what has been hiding beneath the veneer.

The evasive nature of the snake symbolises how difficult Dumuzi is to see in the upperworld. He is camouflaged because he is the norm, the things we accept on the surface that everyone goes along with. To keep spotting these narratives, both at a personal and societal level, is tricky. Seeing and catching Dumuzi takes conscious effort.

Telling the Truth

Dumuzi's charismatic exterior symbolises all the ways we twist the truth to look better on the outside and manipulate things in our favour. It doesn't have to be big lies, it is the day-to-day regularly repeated concealments and omissions that keep our façades in place which make the deepest grooves. These are often so ingrained that half the time we don't even know we are acting them out. There are so many ways that we opt for the socially acceptable version (which usually pertains to masculine energy) of ourselves, whilst sacrificing the truth of our bodies and energy systems. As we rise, we feel the temptation of the old coping strategies. If we want to truly rise, we must put our naked honesty into practice.

I hear people say *"that's my truth"*, which seems to imply that the truth is fixed, *mine,* and absolute. I find that truth is far more nuanced than that. The beauty of truth-telling is that it requires presence. In reality, there are not many absolute truths in life and there can be many truths at play in any given moment. To be tactile to them, we must be in dynamic relationship with ourselves and others, which is what we practice in our rising. The truth appears whilst we are relating. Can we allow the truth to have movement like the snake? Can we allow ourselves the liberation of holding many truths? Where, like Dumuzi, do we disguise or hide from a truth?

Here we encounter another important paradox: hiding or holding something back, does not always mean *not* telling the truth. Some things need time to gestate, some things need protecting. Social media has given rise to a raft of vulnerable reveals and online sharing, where people – mainly women – expose their internal thoughts, feelings and bodies online for all to see. A lesson I have been learning through Inanna is that,

nakedness is not necessarily synonymous with
authenticity, sometimes it is just overexposure.

Part of the compulsion to over-expose myself in the past was born of the desperate need to be seen. As we explored in the last chapter, whilst we are in a dominator dynamic with the masculine, part of us remains invisible, overshadowed by him. Whilst, becoming naked is one route to revelation, wielding 'the sword of truth' of is another. Snakes are also phallic symbols, and part of meeting the snake is about being initiated into the potency of own masculine energy. If we can transform our relationship with our inner masculine, perhaps he can help us to tell the truth in a way that protects us from overexposure. Since I began to feel my inner Dumuzi and he began to work on my behalf, I am less compelled to be naked in situations where I actually need to safeguard myself. When my inner masculine (Dumuzi) grew the capacity to *see* my inner feminine (Inanna), he started to help protect and take care of her. In short,

now I can behold myself, I have less need to over-expose myself.

Desire

Our *eros* is now rising and with it our desire for life. The snake also symbolises our complicated relationship with desire and, in particular, our inherent fear of our own desire. The snake has long been vilified for its role in desire. Most famously, the serpent is the one that tempts Eve to eat the apple. But desire is the pure energy of our life's longing for itself. It is the delight that dances with and directs our *eros* and animates our relationship with all things. So why has desire got such a bad reputation?

As Ereshkigal demonstrates, the shadow side of desire is devouring, vengeance and destruction. The dark side of Dumuzi's desire leads him to dominate and indiscriminately take what he wants. Desire holds power, and when we contact it, it can pull us towards the light, or our shadow. I feel humanity is living in the time of rampant shadow, of devourers and dominators: Ereshkigal and Dumuzi energy. Everything we have tried to exile or ignore – personally and collectively – is now acting out. The Earth's landscapes and increasing temperatures are revealing the costs in ways that are unbearable, almost impossible, to behold.

The Earth is showing us her trauma, and reflecting ours as a species.

The Gorgons were terrifying snake-women in ancient Greek mythology, similar to an Ereshkigal archetype. The most famous of them was Medusa, whose gaze would turn people to stone. She freezes us with fear, an embodied response to stress or trauma. Medusa is said to be so rageful because she was raped, like Ereshkigal, she was traumatised. In the story, Perseus cuts off Medusa's head. If we took a different approach and did not sever her head from her body (like in dissociation), then maybe Medusa could come back into her body and heal. As the Inanna-Ereshkigal myth teaches, when the pain Ereshkigal has been holding is gradually released and reintegrated, the survival energy that has not been able to complete its cycle can be reincarnated. Then the exiled energy can flow unimpeded, with the river of our unfettered life force and natural desires.

If we can gradually access and reintegrate this energy into our nervous system and psychic structures, then the survival response embedded within trauma can catalyse authentic spiritual transformation.

Peter Levine, *In an Unspoken Voice*

Levine's *authentic spiritual transformation* that I feel is embodied in the Inanna-Ereshkigal myth, is so contrary to dualistic dogma, that teaches us that the dark parts of ourselves and our desires must be amputated or suppressed. Traditionally, the Church teaches us that desire is a sin, but in his book *Falling Upward*, Reverend Richard Rohr turns this around,

Losing, falling, failing, sin and the suffering that comes from those experiences – all of this is a necessary and maybe good part of the human journey. As Mother Julian of Norwich said, 'Sin is behovely'. We grow spiritually much more by doing it wrong than by doing it right.

Behovely meaning it is beneficial and actually good for us to sin. In other words, when we *sin* or make mistakes, we learn. If we ride the life force of our desire we will make mistakes, this an inevitable part of rising. So was Eve wrong for eating the apple? Was Inanna bad for going to the underworld? Was Pandora evil for opening the jar? When we eat the apple of self-knowledge, when we descend, when we make mistakes, we grow.

In the Genesis story the serpent is crucial to humankind's journey towards adulthood. Adam and Eve have to be disobedient if they are to journey towards Knowledge and to graduate as full Citizens of the Divine Realm. The Church has been ambivalent about this. In the Easter liturgy the disobedience is called a 'happy sin', a 'felix culpa'. Despite this the Church throughout its

history has not wanted ordinary people to grow up, to enter on an independent
journey towards selfhood – it has oppressed and exiled independent aliveness.
It has kept people immature.

John Hillman

If we do not shame or repress our desire, perhaps we can get to know the map of it and even a desire that is followed 'wrongly' may turn out to be a *felix culpa* that leads us to the most valuable teaching of our lives. Desire itself is not the problem. Returning to the notion of innocence, it is my belief that at the heart of all desire is life. Not good, not bad, just pure life energy. What we do with that, and how we ride the pulsation of it, is what we are learning as we rise.

The word 'desire' derives from the Latin word *desiderare*, which contains within it meanings like "star", "absence of" and "longing for" there are so many echoes of Gate Four here. As Chameli Gad Ardagh teaches,

I love the definition of desire as a feeling of being apart from your star, of
missing your true home, a remembrance of union. Could it be that the tug
from within your heart, that restlessness, and craving, is simply a call from
you to come home? And could it be that your true home is not really a place,
but more like an unfolding, a belonging, an infinite blossoming of being?

What Dumuzi doesn't realise is, that in trying to escape, he is actually avoiding the path that leads home. When we mature into the wisdom of our desire, we develop the understanding that what we think we want, is not always what we need. If we can give up our own arrogant knowing and surrender, we might learn something crucial: as Inanna does when she descends.

> *Let everything into you: Beauty and Terror.*
> *Keep going: remember, no feeling is forever.*
> *Don't lose touch with me.*
> *Nearby is the land*
> *they call Life.*
> *You will recognise it*
> *by its intensity.*
> *Give me your hand.*

from "Before the Beginning" by Rainer Maria Rilke,
translated by Kim Rosen and Maria Krekeler

The Holy Longing

The snake represents fertility and rebirth and conversely, in the shedding of skin, death. The snake has long been a symbol of the Dark Goddess because it embodies the polarities of life and death as a part of its nature. Snake energy teaches us that we can only rebirth ourselves if are willing to relinquish what we have outgrown, or what was never truly ours in the first place.

We must shed our skin.

Unmet desires can become holy longings and the fire inside of our devotion. Can we allow absences and grief to teach, season and transform us? Can we learn to hold the voltage of our unmet longings? Can we allow the creative fire of our longing to build and illuminate things that lie beyond our current understanding?

Journalling exercise on desire

1. Set a timer for 3 minutes and blurt write the same phrase on repeat: *"I desire..."* and see what arises. You may find that one of your desires is really strong, in which case you could write this one over and over again. Or conversely, you may find it hard to fill the time. Everything is valuable information.

2. Then, read through your list and underline ones that you feel devotion to. In my experience, devotion is deeper than our more surface desires. Devotion is desire fuelled with love, passion and sacred commitment. What are you devoted to? Where do your devotions and desires meet?

If you have struggled to contact your desire or devotion this is useful information and may need some more of your attention. Beginning to feel and own our desires is a vital part of our rising fully into aliveness. Notice what has arisen for you in this enquiry.

As we mature, we acquiesce to the truth that some desires cannot – and perhaps even should not – be met. This is to be initiated into holy longing which converts itself into divine creative energy. Longing cultivates the kind of creativity that plumbs the depths and connects us to source. We are moved forwards, one step at a time, through the call inside our longings. Not having, leads us to an infinite well spring of energy that shapes us and our lives in ways that at this point we can only imagine. Longing is the inexhaustible flame inside that will not ever go out: it is the fuel for the artistry of our lives, our creative endeavours, in short, it is an expression of Love.

Love that reaches beyond the personal and into the eternal.

Our most ardent longing is attached to the infinity of all longings. When we discover it, then desire becomes desire for its own sake. It has no final destination, but evolves and shape-shifts through the contours of our lives. If we never dare to meet the snake energy within, we can never touch this, never embody it and never be guided by it.

Embodying the Snake

In yogic practice, the snake represents the kundalini energy in the body, the sleeping life force in the pelvis, that, once awakened, pierces our consciousness and opens us up to spirit. The kundalini energy is said to lay dormant at the base of the spine. When aroused, it rises up *shushumna* (the central channel of the spine) weaving the river that flows between our right and left sides (masculine and feminine) – bringing our polarities into union.

I don't think it's a mistake that many people who have experienced some kind of trauma orientate towards practices like kundalini yoga. If we already have dissociative tendencies, then we will likely be very 'good' at practices which bring the energy up into the higher centres of the body. But if we never descend, these kinds of practices perpetuate our avoidant patterns – which Dumuzi embodies.

As we have explored, many spiritual traditions and practices emphasise the ascent through the chakras. In this book we have reversed the approach because in my experience, *if we focus on the down, the up will see to itself.*

This is what the Inanna story teaches us. It is first the path of downward mobility rather than upwards, which is so contrary to modern, capitalist ideals. In Western culture we are encouraged to be aspirational, to elevate ourselves, get more followers, climb to the top of the pile, constantly tell ourselves we are enough.

We have largely become estranged from the innocence of our desire.

The heroine's journey is the antidote to this. Kundalini the experience, rather than kundalini the brand, is, I have found, a very uncomfortable awakening, that takes us into the underworld of being and those places inside ourselves that have got stuck or are in pain. The snake energy of desire is strong, and it has to be, as it is wrapped up with our desire for life. It is part of our primal survival instinct and urge to procreate. This is why kundalini awakening can be so physically uncomfortable, because if the spinal pathway is impeded by our latent physical and emotional patterns, the energy will have to find another route in our bodies and lives to express itself. As we have seen, it is treacherous territory. The snake of desire can be so powerful that it can kill us. Probably one of the clearest examples of this is in drug addiction, where the part of us that is addicted to the high, will kill, beg, borrow and steal to get its fix. And, in the most extreme outcome, will overdose and be returned to the underworld by the dark side of desire.

As we come back to life, we have to bring consciousness to our desires and chthonic energies, we have to simultaneously awaken to their seductive nature and follow their sacred thread. By walking the gauntlet of our desires, we mature, we learn how to work with the power of the awakened snake energy so it can teach us how to be fully alive. When our *eros* rises, we have the opportunity to embody a new paradigm of partnership, rather than domination. To do this we need to cultivate compassion – the final part of the heroine's journey.

Chapter 15

MEETING GESHTINANNA – COMPASSION AND COMPLETION

Bodhisattva Vows.
Creations are numberless, I vow to free them
Delusions are inexhaustible, I vow to transform them
Reality is boundless, I vow to perceive it
The awakened way is unsurpassable, I vow to embody it.
Let me respectfully remind you,
Life and death are of supreme importance
Time passes swiftly and opportunity is lost
Let us awaken, awaken.
Do not squander your life.

Roshi Joan Halifax

The final character in the myth is Geshtinanna, Dumuzi's sister. Linda Hartley likens her to a Bodhisattva. Bodhisattvas come from the Mahayana Buddhist tradition and are awakened beings that do not transcend to heaven, but instead stay on Earth to help and show compassion for suffering beings. In the Inanna myth, Geshtinanna is the embodiment of this wisdom. She is another aspect of the witness, the part within us that can bear to be with all of our complexity. She can behold our fear and encourages us to move forwards in spite of it. In the story, she is the one that Dumuzi appeals to for help and she feels deeply for his troubles.

Geshtinanna appeals to Inanna to have mercy on Dumuzi and offers to sacrifice herself and take his place in the underworld. As Linda Hartley expounds, *Geshtinanna's offer is not the martyrdom of a woman who cannot stand her own ground and gives herself away out of false motives; she offers herself out of her deep love for her brother in his suffering. Geshtinanna is a woman of wisdom, a seer, a prophetess.*

Inanna's own grief and loving consciousness is magnetised to the surface though Geshtinanna's offering. Without Geshtinanna, Inanna may have acted out the sacrifice of Dumuzi from an unconscious, vengeful place, like when Ereshkigal enacted her wrath on Inanna. In this case, there is a danger that our Dumuzi aspect (the inner masculine) would be amputated and lost in the underworld. With Geshtinanna's presence Inanna can become the initiatress of Dumuzi. Compassion is vital if we are to consciously integrate the teachings of the descent and rise without splitting, losing or exiling any part of ourselves at this last crucial moment.

With compassion, Inanna is able to find a compromise that is aligned with her integrity and the laws of the underworld. She decrees that Geshtinanna will go to the underworld for half the year and then Dumuzi must descend for other half of the year. Both the masculine (Dumuzi) and feminine (Geshtinanna) within us must be initiated. Geshtinanna is the sister whose love bridges the gap between our dualities. If we are to sit within the complexity of our experience and accept that we cannot transcend the paradoxes within, we need Geshtinanna to awaken within us. She embodies the cultivation of our capacity to be deeply loving towards all of our vulnerabilities and contradictions. She is our essential ability to hold nuance and pendulate between the heights and the depths.

Gifts of Emergence

When I spoke to women about their own descents a question I asked was, *"what was the gift that you have emerged with?"* And the answer was almost always the same: women referred to a broader capacity to be with themselves and others in their pain. Compassion seems to be the thing that our heroine's journey cultivates within us. Returning to Jacinta Meteur's story, she spoke to how her descent helped her become a Geshtinanna within the S.H.E. College Fund for other girls,

"I can really see the impact for now almost twenty years, I have seen big transformation in my life and I have learned a lot. I have seen many people change in that period. When I finished primary school, I didn't have a role model. But I was lucky that I was able to struggle on my own...I struggled a lot and that helped me to get stronger. So working for S.H.E., I can really understand or relate to the girls' situations. I can notice who needs more care, in terms of mentorship, in terms of counselling, in terms of just talking to them, encouraging them. So I am able to understand and help them and mentor them and notice who needs help. Because when I look at their backgrounds, I can relate to their situation. In terms of my patience and being available for them all the time, that's really helped me help them. Because it's a situation that I went through, so I understand it."

Sophie Jane Hardy also articulated it in a way that really resonated with me,

"I can now actually sit with people in their pain, and I don't think I could before. I notice that when people used to bring pain to me, I used to share something about myself as a way to try to say, 'I am in pain too, we can do this together'. But I now know that that is not how it's always received. What I realise now is that when someone brings pain to me, I don't have do anything except be with them. So that's been a huge gift of this experience. I can be with pain, more in myself, but with others especially."

Geshtinanna is the willingness to be with our own suffering and that of others rather than turn away. She is the one who has the generosity to be with what feels difficult, even impossible at times, and stay present, with love. She helps us yield to our resistance and integrate what we are grieving with what is being birthed. For me, she stands for an emotional integrity that can only come through adversity and maturity. Her presence is absolutely crucial, if we are to truly discover the wisdom of our trauma.

The Life/Death/Life of Natural Cycles

Geshtinanna is the presence that helps us complete our cycles. The myth in its entirety holds an embodied teaching of cyclical wisdom. Geshtinanna is the part of us that has compassion for our addictions, avoidant strategies, fear and human fallibility. She helps Dumuzi find the courage and compassion to surrender so that he can uncover the Enki within. She grounds us in cyclical wisdom and the laws of nature, which includes the base notes, the emptiness, the death, the fallow parts of the cycle.

One of my avoidant strategies is rushing and trying to do it all. When the Geshtinanna part of me can open to the feelings underneath my rushing, I can experience the pain/vulnerability that lies underneath my addiction to speed and stimulation. From this part of myself, I have experienced genuine sorrow for the ways I have hurt myself, the ways I have been my own slave driver and the ways that I have hurt others. Be that allowing life to become so busy that I am emotionally unavailable for my kids, my avoidance of sensual pleasure when it is what I most need and cannot give it to myself, or in being too 'generous' with my time, money, and what I shoulder, at the expense of myself – all these are forms of self-abandonment. Compassion interrupts the habit of self-abandonment.

Back Down to Earth

Since the spirit of our times is based on linear growth, domination and ascent, I would argue that cyclical wisdom, partnership and descent are the soulful practices to counter that.

Something to bring us back down to Earth.

The protagonist of all our stories is actually the Earth. She is the one from whose story we cannot separate.

When I land into my body, into nature and what is underneath our human world, I contact the pain and shame of the destruction that we are wreaking on the Earth. I struggle to be compassionate to this side of our humanity and the ways that I am complicit with it. When I recognise the magnitude of our human catastrophe it feels unbearable. Being compassionate does not mean saying that everything we do is okay if it is not. If compassion is the willingness to suffer with, then we have to be willing to feel the reality and consequences of our actions. Not just turn our heads the other way. This teaching from Indigenous activist Lyla June really broke my heart open,

We belong on the land. We belong in active participation with the land. Without our gentle, loving and reciprocal touch, our clipping, burning, pruning and manicuring, our mother falls apart. Just look at the pine beetles ripping through our national park forests. Just look at the catastrophic fires gobbling up lands where our light indigenous fires used to clear the light fuel load every single season for thousands of years. The Earth needs us. Do you really think creator would make humans without purpose? In the Yoruba language they call humans 'the chosen ones', because they were chosen to take care of and steward the land. This is why it aches so deeply to see our Mother Earth crumble all around us. To see coyote destroy ancient systems, to see coyote hijack our greed and fear to do so. Because deep down in the marrow of our bones we know we were created to care for her [...] Here we are poised ready to take it back again. Take back our mantel and our role as Earth stewards.

For a long time my overriding feeling towards humanity has been shame because of our relationship to the Earth. But this turned me back towards our place within the ecosystem, where our interbeing can be in service of the Earth.

Is it too late to pick up that mantle of 'earth steward' again?

It can feel impossible to think of one big solution to the situation we have created. I wonder if there is a rightness in this too. Because big monocultures, big business that removes us from community and biodiversity, is, as I see it, a huge part of the problem. So we have to start small, from the ground up, we must address the personal.

What we are standing on in the personal and collective, always, is the edge of the labyrinth of life, the unknown. The story begins with Inanna opening her ears to the Great Below. At the beginning her understanding is limited, just as at this point, so is ours. Diane Wolkstein speaks about how in Sumerian, the word for ear and wisdom is the same. The inner ear is coiled like the spiral of a labyrinth. When we open to listening to the depths, we may be able to translate what we hear from imperceptible sound, to an understanding of new meaning that guides our actions.

I would sell my tongue and buy a thousand ears when that one steps near to speak.

Rumi

When we begin to consciously honour and re-connect to cyclical living and the Earth, it can feel as though we are speaking a different language that no one will understand. How do we trust the discomfort that comes with these transitions? Can we stay with them long enough to learn how to live congruently in the upperworld? At first, we don't know how and, what's more, we cannot rely on our old coping mechanisms to find out. So, in a sense, we continue to walk with underworld feet above ground and we leave footprints of Ereshkigal's wisdom everywhere we go. We keep learning, we are never done. With Geshtinanna's presence we can descend and rise as many times as necessary, to reveal the lessons we need to learn.

CLOSING

I would not sacrifice my Soul
for all the beauty of this world,
There is only one thing
for which I would risk everything,
That, "And I don't know what"
that lies in the heart of the mystery.
The taste of finite pleasure leads nowhere.
All is does is exhaust the appetite and ravage the palate.
So I would not sacrifice my Soul
for all the sweetness of this world.
But I would risk everything
for that "I don't know what"
that lives at the heart of the mystery.

from "Glosa a lo Divino" in Saint John of the Cross,
translated by Mirabai Starr

Inanna teaches us that we cannot seek the Great Above without connection to the Great Below. A core theme of this myth is about going towards our shadow to discover its essence – our light.

The heroine's path can be a lonely road, but if we have the courage to stay with it, little by little, we start to attract other heroines towards us, creating new communities and webs of connection.

Together we weave a different narrative, hopefully one that honours the Earth more and more. I have heard so many people I work with say, *"I don't fit in with that social group anymore"* or *"I feel like I have changed and the world has stayed the same".* Walking in integrity means necessary loss, but the final part of the journey also heralds a renewal of our sense of interbeing. The stories we tell help shape our world and the stories we live even more so. Stories can become armour that protects us for a time, but then weighs us down and keeps us separated.

What I love most about the Inanna-Ereshkigal myth is that it is about taking the armour off, by disrupting the stories entrenched within and exposing us to what we have not previously been able to see, or feel. In this fragile time of populism and polarisation, it feels essential that we become more intimate with the Sky Gods, the Ninshubur, the Ereshkigal, the Dumuzi, the Enki, the Geshtinanna and the Inanna within, so that we might truly get to touch our own nakedness and the nakedness of others – the place where, even if only for a moment, we connect. As the old stories die, we become tactile to a sixth sense that guides us forwards, no longer functioning from defensiveness, but from our vulnerability and presence. And everything that seemed broken, shameful, dark and irreparable is transformed. Not necessarily healed – but the journey changes the way we fit into the ecosystem.

The heroine's journey is an erotic, mystical initiation that revivifies *our place in the shape of things.* [*]

The fodder of our descents provides the compost from which the richest fruits of our lives can grow. If only we can turn towards our pain and let it work in us. This myth consecrated my descent, it sanctified the journey as a heroine's initiation, rather than just a failure or break down.

I was Inanna.

And this was what I learned through my descent and rising.

You, too are Inanna. You can choose to descend, dare to reach your roots back down into the Earth, so that you can rise back up into the upperworld embodying something ancient and new.

* Albert Huffstickler

DESCENT & RISING

The dark cocoon of heartbreak is vital ground.
Through that devastated shipwreck appear the wings of spirit.
The second birth canal,
whose rivers deliver us back to the heart of it all.
In the ruthless light of day,
one bridge burns,
and we are no longer our Fathers' daughters.
The stretcher we wake up on carries us,
through the thickets of the soul towards a new beyond.
Heartbreak for one
becomes a grieving for the whole world.
Our embryonic heartbeats compel us to build new bridges,
bridges that hum to the song.
We remember,
and our footsteps touch the ground tenderly in their authority.
The bridge to the Goddess is built through a sincere heart,
and no heart is more sincere,
than that of the unwitting warrior who has found her yes,
who cannot possibly remain folded.
That one, who through being broken in two
is delivered back into one with everything.

CONTRIBUTOR BIOGRAPHIES

(In order of appearance.) Please note that not all contributors are listed here, as some chose to contribute using a pseudonym.

Angela Farmer has been practicing and teaching yoga since 1965 and is known across the world for her unique and innovative approach, a process where tradition and style are replaced by a personal journey, guided by one's own inner wisdom, intuition and a profound relationship with nature, to find truth, freedom and joy in living. She and her husband Victor Van Kooten live and teach on the Greek island of Lesvos. angela-victor.com

Trista Hendren founded Girl God Books in 2011 to support a necessary unravelling of the patriarchal world view of divinity. Her first book – *The Girl God,* a children's picture book – was a response to her own daughter's inability to see herself reflected in God. Since then, she has published more than forty books by a dozen women from across the globe. Originally from Portland, Oregon, she now lives in Bergen, Norway with her family. thegirlgod.com

Sivani Mata is a UK born and bred artist who is moved by a sensory and elemental exploration of life through practice that evokes the liminal experience of trance-like states of consciousness (such as Kirtan and Yoga Nidra) as a way to cultivate a harmonic relationship with the Earth, and to build the relationship of self-love and acceptance. She is currently writing a book called *Faces of the Feminine* exploring the feminine sacred in different cultures around the world. naturalmysticbhajans.co.uk

Priscilla Rodgers is an embodiment coach based in California. She has created a method to guide women back into living fully, unapologetically and sensuously in their bodies. She works with women one-on-one and in group settings using a form of body-centered meditation she calls a Sensescape. She has also recently become passionate about childhood trauma and how it holds us back from living a fully embodied life.

Sophie Jane Hardy is a nature- and cycle-inspired business coach, writer and podcast host, currently living by the River Rivelin in Sheffield, UK with her husband, son, and dog. Her work has evolved over a decade of non-profit communications, documentary filmmaking, women's leadership and environmental activism. She is the creator of the "Your Cyclical Business" online programme and the host of The Menstruality Podcast. sophiejanehardy.com

Dawn Oakley-Smith is a practitioner of Equine Facilitated Human Development with twenty years' experience. She runs HeartShore Horses in the Cotswolds. As well as EFHD, a large part of her work is guiding groups of people through shamanic processes such as Horse Dancing and Soul Recognition. Accompanied by her herd of eighteen horses, and with poetry and meditative practices, participants are held and guided on their journeys to the underworld to find release and healing. heartshore-horses.co.uk

Lucy H. Pearce is the author of many life-changing non-fiction books, including Nautilus Award winners *Medicine Woman, Burning Woman,* and *Creatrix: she who makes.* Lucy is a multi-faceted creative whose work spans the expressive arts, exploring the lost archetypes of the feminine. Lucy founded Womancraft Publishing, publishing paradigm-shifting books by women for women, in 2014. A mother of three, she lives in East Cork, Ireland. lucyhpearce.com

Kalia Wright is a Shadow Integration guide and certified Psychosexual Somatics coach currently living at Osho Leela in Dorset. Kalia is devoted to serving embodied truth, wholeness and integrity in herself and others. She works with people to compassionately dismantle blocks to being fully expressed in life. Kalia has evolved her practice from over ten years of child protection social work and over seventeen years of personal and spiritual development, including an MSc in Psychology. kaliawright.com

Jacinta Silantoi Meteur earned her BS in Business, and went on to get an MBA in Business Administration in Kenya. Her passion to attend college compelled her to reach out to Kim Rosen for help in 2010, and their collaboration in her college education was the seed that became the S.H.E Fund. She is now the Director of Kenya Operations for the S.H.E. College Fund. shecollegefund.org

Tamara Albanna is a writer, artist, Reiki healer, and Tarot reader. In 2012, while researching her Master's thesis on her motherland Iraq, she became reacquainted with Inanna and travelled to the underworld. She has since written extensively about the Divine Feminine. tamara-albanna.com

REFERENCES

Opening

Wolkstein, Diane and Kramer, Samuel. *Inanna: Queen of Heaven and Earth,* Harper and Row Publishers, New York, 1983.

Hartley, Linda. *Servants of the Sacred Dream: Rebirthing the Deep Feminine: Psycho-Spiritual Crisis and Healing,* Elmdon Books, Norfolk, 2001

Lauter, Estella. *Women as Mythmakers: Poetry and Visual Art by Twentieth-Century Women,* Indiana University Press, Indiana, 1984

Chapter 1 – The Heroine's Journey

Wolkstein, Diane and Kramer, Samuel. *Inanna: Queen of Heaven and Earth,*

1. pp.58-9
2. pp.64-65
3. p.66
4. p.69
5. p.89

Chapter 2

Bly, Robert. "You Darkness, that I come from" from *Selected Poems of Rainer Maria Rilke, A Translation from the German and Commentary by Robert Bly.* Copyright © 1981 by Robert Bly.

Carter, Sue. *The Biology of Love,* The Kinsey Institute Indiana University, Indiana, 2020 therapistuncensored.com/wp-content/uploads/2020/09/The-Kinsey-Institute-ebook-Feb-20-V4-8449.pdf

Murdock, Maureen. *The Heroine's Journey,* Shambala Publications Inc., Boulder Colorado, 1990, p.89

Owen, Lara. *Her Blood is Gold,* Archive Publishing, 2008, p. xv

Oliver, Mary. Excerpt of "Wild Geese" in *New and Selected Poems Vol.1,* Beacon Press, Boston, 1992

Pinkola Estés, Clarissa. *Women Who Run with the Wolves,* Random House, London, 1992, p.1

Jung, Carl, Gustav. *The Red Book: A Reader's Edition* Edited by S. Shamdasani
W.W. Norton and Company, New York and London, 2001, p.129

Chapter 3

Levine, Peter. *In An Unspoken Voice: How the Body Releases Trauma and Restores Goodness,* North Atlantic Books, Berkeley, 2010, p.35

Maté, Gabor. Quote taken from an online course, "The Role of Spiritual Awakening in Trauma Healing", "The Trauma and Awakening Programme" with Dr Gabor Maté and Alex Howard. Video 1, 2021 trauma.consciouslife.com/videos/

Rothschild, Babette. *The Body Remembers – The Psychophysiology of Trauma and Trauma Treatment,* W.W. Norton and Company, New York and London, 2000

Van Der Kolk, Bessel. *The Body Keeps the Score: Mind, Brain and Body in the Transformation of Trauma,* Penguin, London, 2015

Johnson, Kimberly Ann. *The Call of the Wild,* Harper Wave, New York, 2021, p.24

Porges, Stephen. *The Polyvagal Theory Neurophysiological Foundations of Emotions, Attachment, Communication and Self-Regulation,* W.W Norton and Company, New York and London, 2011

Levine, Peter. *In An Unspoken Voice,* p.99

Weller, Francis. *The Wild Edge of Sorrow,* North Atlantic Books, 2012, p.8

Chapter 4

Christ, Carol. *Diving Deep and Surfacing,* Beacon Press, Boston, 1980, p.1

Eisler, Riane. *The Chalice and the Blade: Our History, Our Future,* Harper San Francisco, San Francisco, 1988, p.xix

Reuther, Rosemary. *Goddesses and the Divine Feminine: A Western Religious History,* University of California Press, 2005, p, 284

Condren, Mary. "On Forgetting Our Divine Origins: The Warnings of Dervogilla", *Irish Journal of Feminist Studies* vol. 2 no. 1: 117-132, 1997
academia.edu/4873730/ON_FORGETTING_OUR_DIVINE_ORIGINS_THE_WARNING_OF_DERVOGILLA

Nicholson, Sarah. *The Evolutionary Journey of Woman,* The Neo Perennial Press, 2016, p.12

Murdock, Maureen. *The Heroine's Journey,* p.1

Lorde, Audre. "The Master's Tools Will Never Dismantle the Master's House", *The Selected Works of Audre Lorde,* W.W. Norton and Company, Inc., New York, 2020, p. 41

Pinkola Estés, Clarissa. *Women Who Run with the Wolves,* p.376

International Pathwork Foundation. "The Idealized Self-Image – Pathwork Guide Lecture No. 83", 1961, pathwork.org/lectures/the-idealized-self-image

Chapter 5

Woodman, Marion and Dickson, Elinor. *Dancing in the Flames – The Dark Goddess in the Transformation of Consciousness,* Shambala Publications, Boulder Colorado, 1997, p.21

Wolkstein, Diane and Kramer, Samuel. *Inanna: Queen of Heaven and Earth,* p.56

Hardwicke Collings, Jane. *Herstory* janehardwickecollings.com/wp-content/uploads/2018/04/herstory_ebook.pdf 2008, pp.14-5

Lerner, Gerda. (ed) "The Creation of Feminist Consciousness: From the Middle Ages to Eighteen-seventy", Oxford University Press, 1994

Awakening Women. awakeningwomen.com

Miller, Madeline. *Circe,* Bloomsbury Publishing, London, 2022

Favilli, Elena and Cavallo, Francesca. *Goodnight Stories for Rebel Girls: 100 tales of extraordinary women,* Particular Books, London, 2017

D'Addario, Daniel, Nathan, Giri and Rayman, Noah. "The 100 Best Children's Books of All Time", *TIME Magazine,* 2016, time.com/100-best-childrens-books/

Davis, Geena. Quote cited from "The Geena Davis Institute on Gender in Media" website, 2022, seejane.org/about-us

Christ, Carol. Quote cited in Diane Stein's anthology *The Goddess Celebrates,* Crossing Press, Canada, 1991, p.253

Chapter 6

Brinton Perera, Sylvia. *The Descent to the Goddess A Way of Initiation,* Inner City Books, Toronto, 1981, p.63

Hartley, Linda. *Servants of the Sacred Dream,* p.162

Coel, Michaela. "I May Destroy You", British television programme created, written, co-directed and produced by Michaela Coel for the BBC and HBO, 2021

The Descent

Rosen, Kim. Excerpt from "Autobiography of 1994", kimrosen.net

Gate 1

Wolkstein, Diane and Kramer, Samuel. *Inanna: Queen of Heaven and Earth,* p.58

Rosen, Kim. *Saved By a Poem: The Transformative Power of Words,* p.157

Murdock, Maureen. *The Heroine's Journey,* Shambala Publications, Boulder Colorado, 1990, p.84

Hartley, Linda. *Servants of the Sacred Dream,* p.159

Blackie, Sharon. "The Mythic Feminine and the Post-Heroic Journey". Interview on 'The Knitted Heart Podcast', Episode 8, 2020 knittedheart.com/podcast/sharonblackie

Judith, Anodea. *Eastern Body Western Mind,* Random House, New York, 2004, p.393

Gate 2

Pearce, Lucy, H. *Burning Woman,* Womancraft Publishing, Cork, 2016, p.46

Gate 3

Zwicky, Jan. Excerpt from "The Art of Fugue: VI" in Forge, Gaspereau Press, Canada, 2019

Rosen, Kim. *Saved By a Poem,* p.165, p.154

Porges, Stephen. "Embodiment Through the Lens of the Polyvagal Theory". The Embodiment Conference interview, 2020 portal.theembodimentconference.org/sessions/embodiment-through-the-lens-of-the-polyvagal-theory-5c1ic8

Bryant, Olivia. Self Cervix selfcervix.com

Beard, Mary. *Women and Power – A Manifesto,* Profile Books, London, 2017, p.4, p.41

Bates, Laura. "Everyday Sexism" TED Talk, 2013 www.ted.com/talks/laura_bates_everyday_sexism?language=en

Johnson, Kimberly Ann. *The Call of the Wild: How We Heal Trauma, Awaken Our Own Power and Use It for Good,* Harperwave, 2021

La Rosa, Sarah. "The Voice You Thought You Lost". sarahlarosa.com

Gate 4

Oliver, Mary. Excerpt from "Sunrise" in *New and Selected Poems Vol.1,* Beacon Press, Boston, 1992, p.125

Pinkola Estés, Clarrissa. *Untie The Strong Woman: Immaculate Mothers Love for the Wild Soul,* Sounds True, Colorado, 2013, p.78-79

Reilly, Patricia Lynn. *Be Full of Yourself: The Journey from Self-Criticism to Self-Celebration,* Open Window Creations, 1998

Tempest, Kae. *On Connection,* Faber, London, 2020, p.34

Weller, Francis. *The Wild Edge of Sorrow,* p.4

Kunitz, Stanley. Excerpt from "The Layers" in *The Collected Poems of Stanley Kunitz,* W.W Norton & Company, New York, 2002

Tweedy, Irina. *Daughter of Fire – A Diary of a Spiritual Training with a Sufi Master,* The Golden Sufi Center, 1986, p.v

Jimenez, Juan Ramon. Excerpt from "'I Am Not I'" in *Lorca and Jiménez: Selected Poems,* 1973 by Robert Bly. Beacon Press, 1973

Cope, Stephen. *The Great Work of Your Life,* Random House, 2012, p.254

Eisler, Riane. *The Chalice and the Blade: Our History, Our Future,* p.20

Gate 5

Twitchell, Chase. Excerpt from "Saint Animal" in *The Snow Watcher*, W.W. Norton & Company, Inc., New York, 2013

Rilke, Rainer Maria. Excerpt from "Dedication", original translation and source unknown.

Bairstow, Cedar. *Living in the Power Zone: the right use of power can transform your relationships*, Many Realms Press, 2013, p.20

Jung, Carl, Gustav. *The Red Book*, p.73

Condren, Mary. "On Forgetting Our Divine Origins: The Warnings of Dervogilla", *Irish Journal of Feminist Studies vol. 2 no. 1: 117-132*, 1990

hooks, bell. *All About Love*, Harper Perennial, 2001

McGilchrist, Ian. *The Matter with Things: Our Brains, Our Delusions, and the Unmaking of the World*, Perspectiva, 2021

Gate 6

Kabir. "I talk to my inner lover" from *The Kabir Book Versions* by Robert Bly, 1977, p.23

Heavens, Jules. Personal conversation quoted with permission from Jules Heavens, 2022, julesheavens.com

Pope, Alexandra and Hugo-Wurlitzer, Sjanie. *Wild Power*, Hay House, 2017, p.45

Tedlock, Barbara. *The Woman in the Shaman's Body*, Random House, New York, 2005, p.198

Kramer, Henricus. and Sprenger, Jacobus. *Malleus Maleficarium*, Dover, New York, 1971, p.47

Pinkola Estés, Clarissa. *Women Who Run with the Wolves*, p.413

Wolkstein, Diane and Kramer, Samuel. *Inanna: Queen of Heaven and Earth*, p.37

Judith, Anodea. *Eastern Body Western Mind*, p.121

Lorde, Audre. "Uses of the Erotic: The Erotic as Power" (1978) in *The Selected Works of Audre Lorde*, W.W. Norton and Co, New York, 2021, p.29

Wolfe, Aisha. Excerpt from "Dear Woman" in *Yoniverse Burlesque*, Emerging Now Press, 2013

Gate 7

V. *The Vagina Monologues*, Virago, 1996

Fairchild, Edveejee. Excerpt from "The Roots of a Woman" in *When You Were Forest and Moonlight Complete Edition*, 2019

Murdock, Maureen. *The Heroine's Journey*, 1990 p.155-156

Dinsmore-Tuli, Uma. *Yoni Shakti*, Yogawords Ltd, London, 2014

Eisler, Riane. *The Chalice and the Blade*

Rilke, Rainer Maria. Excerpt from "The Departure of the Prodigal Son" translated by Kim Rosen, 2020.

Wardere, Hibo. "Cut: One Woman's Fight Against FGM In Britain Today," Simon and Schuster, United Kingdom, 2016

Christian Anderson, H. "The Emperor's New Clothes" in *Fairy Tales Told for Children,* C.A Reitzel, Copenhagen, 1837

Pareyio, Agnes. "Rising to End FGM", article on One Billion Rising Website, 2022 onebillionrising.org/27-many-also-sign-revolution-agnes-pareyio

The Underworld

Wolkstein, Diane and Kramer, Samuel. *Inanna: Queen of Heaven and Earth,* p.60

Chapter 8

Hartley, Linda. *Servants of the Sacred Dream,* p.163

Rilke, Rainer Maria. Excerpt from "The Man Watching" in *Selected Poems of Rainer Maria Rilke: A Translation from the German and Commentary* by Robert Bly, Harper Perennial, New York, 1981, p.105

Gangaji. "The Courage to Give Up Hope". Gangaji Radio podcast online, 2016 gangaji. org/gf-podcast/courage-to-give-up-hope

Ostaseski, Frank. *The Five Invitations,* Flatiron Books, 2017, p.1

Chapter 9

Albanna, Tamara and Hendren, Trista. *Inanna's Ascent: Reclaiming Female Power* Girl God Books, 2018, p.2

Lorde, Audre. "The Uses of Anger: Women Responding to Racism", 1981 blackpast.org/ african-american-history/1981-audre-lorde-uses-anger-women-responding-racism

Johnson, Kimberly Ann. *The Call of the Wild,* p.119, p.220, p.125

Chapter 11

Pinkola Estés, Clarissa. *Women Who Run with the Wolves,* 1988

Ardagh, Chameli. "The Fierce Face of the Feminine", Ted Talk, 2016 youtube.com/ watch?v=dcDCXzX_HQA

Wolkstein, Diane and Kramer, Samuel. *Inanna: Queen of Heaven and Earth*

Brinton Perera, Sylvia. *The Descent to the Goddess,* p.67

Jenkinson, Stephen. Sex, Birth, Trauma podcast hosted by Kimberly Ann Johnson, kimberlyannjohnson.com/podcasts, 2021

Strand, Sophie. *The Flowering Wand: Rewilding the Sacred Masculine,* Inner Traditions, 2022

Rising – The Ascent

Adams, MJ. "Turning", 2012

Chapter 12

Hartley, Linda. *Servants of the Sacred Dream*, p.171

Hall, Nor. *The Moon and the Virgin*, Harper Collins, Glasgow, 1980

Gimbutas, Maria. *The Civilisation of the Goddess*, Thorsons Publishers, London, 1991, p.223

Qualls-Corbett, Nancy. *The Sacred Prostitute: Eternal Aspect of the Feminine*, Inner City Books, Toronto, 1988

Howe, M. "Annunciation", 2008

Woodman, Marion. *The Pregnant Virgin: A Process of Psychological Transformation*, Inner City Books, Toronto, 1985

Merton, Thomas. *Conjectures of a Guilty Bystander*, Penguin Random House online excerpt, 1968, earthandspiritcenter.org/wp-content/uploads/2019/10/Session-8-5-Le-Point-Vierge.pdf

Wolkstein, Diane and Kramer, Samuel. *Inanna: Queen of Heaven and Earth*, p.68

Chapter 13

Bates, Laura. *Fix the System, Not the Women*, Simon and Schuster, UK, 2022

Adshead, Gwen. Changes podcast hosted by Annie Macmanus, anniemacmanus.com/changes-podcast/dr-gwen-adshead, 2022

Chapter 14

Cirlot, Juan. *A Dictionary of Symbols* translated from the Spanish by Jack Sage. Routledge, London, 1969, online source, ia801306.us.archive.org/9/items/DictionaryOfSymbols/Dictionary%20of%20Symbols.pdf p.285

Levine, Peter. *In An Unspoken Voice*

Rohr, Richard. *Falling Upward: A Spirituality for the Two Halves of Life*, Jossey Bass, Hoboken, NJ, 2021

Hillman, John. Quote taken from personal email, included with permission from John Hillman, johnhillman.org, 2021

Ardagh, Chameli. Quote taken from @chameliardagh Instagram post, used with permission from Chameli Ardagh, 2022

Rilke, Rainer Maria. Excerpt from "Before the Beginning" translated by Kim Rosen and Maria Krekeler. From the audio recording, Only Breath, Out Front Music, 2007

Chapter 15

Halifax, Joan. *Bodhisattva Vows spoken on Upaya Dharma Course with Roshi Joan Halifax and Frank Ostaseski*. Printed with permission from Roshi Joan Halifax, 2021

upaya.org

Hartley, Linda. *Servants of the Sacred Dream*, p.177

June, Lyla. lylajune.com, 2022

Wolkstein, Diane and Kramer, Samuel. *Inanna: Queen of Heaven and Earth*, p.156

Rumi, Jelaluddin. Excerpt from "Listening" from *The Glance*, translated by Coleman Barks, Penguin, New York, 2001, p. 90

Closing

John of the Cross, "Glosa a lo Divino" in *Saint John of the Cross: Luminous Darkness*, *trans*. Mirabai Starr, Albuquerque, New Mexico: CAC Publishing, 2022, pp.73-75

Huffstickler, Albert. "The Cure" in *Walking Wounded*, Backyard Press, 1989

ACKNOWLEDGEMENTS

To all the women in this book who, like Inanna, became naked and allowed their story to become a teaching. I am so grateful for your courage, trust and words. And to Jo Farrington for kindly sharing some of your experiences of Butterfly. Also to the women who shared their stories with me that I did not manage to include, Muna Mcadie, Aki Omori, Louise Manzanti and Pam England, your presence helped shape this book – thank you.

To Sophie Jane Hardy, for your presence and encouraging me to reach out into new landscapes of marketing in a joyful way.

To Meike Hakkaart, for the powerful cover art.

To Libby Kerr, for helping me hold my client work alongside my writing.

To all the poets, teachers and writers whose words and work are woven through this book and who have supported me in my own heroine's journey. And especially to Diane Wolkstein and Samuel Kramer, for their translation of Enheduanna's mythology.

To Chameli Ardagh and the Awakening Women Wisdom School, for your embodied teachings and sadhanas, especially the beautiful Inanna Sadhana.

To Linda Hartley, whose writing led me to Inanna, and whose wisdom and retreats offered me sustenance, insight and holding in the depths, and in my rising.

To my publisher Lucy H. Pearce, whose edits were inspired and mysteriously synchronistic. Your presence as the Ninshubur of this book has been utterly invaluable. And also to Leigh, Patrick and Sarah at Womancraft Publishing, for your creativity and helping to bring the book into being.

To all the people I have worked with, past and present, and special thanks to the all the Butterflies who have travelled into the landscapes of the wild feminine with me. You bring me heart and hope.

To Lucy Tierney, for being a reader and a soul friend. And to all my friends in the Poetry Depths Mystery and Breathwork community, thank you for giving me a spiritual community to rest into and a space to be naked and unashamed.

To Jules Heavens, for being my Ninshubur, for introducing me to the seasons of the menstrual cycle, and for feminine wisdom and holding.

To John Hillman, for being my Enki. For your unconditional love, for your support when I got stuck in my writing, and for introducing me to poetry.

Meeting you changed my life.

To my Teacher, Kim Rosen, this work would not exist in the way that it does without your teaching, mentorship and love. Thank you for holding me as I dissolved in the cocoon, and celebrating me as I spread my wings and for the gift of Breathwork. So grateful to have you in my life.

To all the fabulous women in my life with special mention to, Cordelia, for a lasting friendship that was a saving grace for me in the underworld and whilst forming Butterfly. To Kate, for all the walks, talks, new moons, sharing motherhood and being a true friend. And to my oldest friends, Anna, Caitlin, Polly and Donna, for being constants in my life over so many years.

To Frances and Mowbray, thank you for always being so supportive and for welcoming me into your family.

To my grandparents, I feel so grateful to have known all four of you. Special thanks to my grandma to who this book is dedicated. And to my nannan, 100 years old and still sparkling, what a woman.

To my brother Luke, for growing with me.

To my parents, for questioning narratives and teaching me to do the same. To my mum, for giving birth to me, for starting me dancing and always encouraging me to follow what makes me happy. To my dad, for your creative and unconventional ways that taught me not to be afraid to be different. And for all the Madonna concerts! Thank you both for everything. I am very grateful for all my family and friends.

To my husband, James, for being the most loyal, supportive, passionate and loving partner I could possibly wish for. For trusting the underworld journey and being there beside me through it. Not many men have the generosity and courage that you have. I love you.

To my daughters, for being my greatest teachers and inspiration. Special thanks to Aurora, for creating the spiral map of the heroine's journey and the snake icons. And to Mimi, for drawing the Inanna-Ereshkigal map of the menstrual cycle. There aren't words enough to express how much I love you both.

And to Inanna, Ereshkigal, Enheduanna and the depths of the mystery and the Earth that holds us all. May we remember.

INDEX

ABOUT THE AUTHOR

Carly Mountain is a women's initiatory guide, a psychotherapist, a psychosexual somatic therapist, yoga teacher, breathworker and writer. For the last twenty years she has worked with sacred embodied practices. Carly stumbled across the Inanna story during her own descent to the underworld and was astonished by the symmetry it held with her own lived experience. Since then she has devoted to working with the myth and specialises in beholding others as they traverse the depths of initiation; both in therapy, breathwork 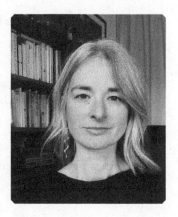 and within courses that support women's awakening and unfolding.

In 2019 Carly self-published her first poetry pamphlet *Jouissance: Poetry of the Deep Feminine. Descent & Rising: Women's Stories and the Embodiment of the Inanna Myth* is Carly's debut non-fiction book. She lives in Sheffield, England with her husband and two daughters.

ABOUT THE ARTIST

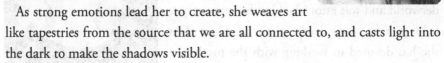

ArtofMaquenda/Meike Hakkaart is an artist living in the Netherlands, drawn to the wild, weird and wonderful aspects of life.

With a passion for nature and a fascination for the cycles of life, she incorporates this childlike curiosity into her work.

As strong emotions lead her to create, she weaves art like tapestries from the source that we are all connected to, and casts light into the dark to make the shadows visible.

ABOUT WOMANCRAFT

Womancraft Publishing was founded on the revolutionary vision that women and words can change the world. We act as midwife to transformational women's words that have the power to challenge, inspire, heal and speak to the silenced aspects of ourselves.

We believe that:

- books are a fabulous way of transmitting powerful transformation,

- values should be juicy actions, lived out,

- ethical business is a key way to contribute to conscious change.

At the heart of our Womancraft philosophy is fairness and integrity. Creatives and women have always been underpaid. Not on our watch! We split royalties 50:50 with our authors. We work on a full circle model of giving and receiving: reaching backwards, supporting TreeSisters' reforestation projects, and forwards via Worldreader, providing books at no cost to education projects for girls and women.

We are proud that Womancraft is walking its talk and engaging so many women each year via our books and online. Join the revolution! Sign up to the mailing list at womancraftpublishing.com and find us on social media for exclusive offers:

 womancraftpublishing

 womancraft_publishing

 womancraftpublishing.com/books

USE OF WOMANCRAFT WORK

Often women contact us asking if and how they may use our work. We love seeing our work out in the world. We love you sharing our words further. And we ask that you respect our hard work by acknowledging the source of the words.

We are delighted for short quotes from our books – up to 200 words – to be shared as memes or in your own articles or books, provided they are clearly accompanied by the author's name and the book's title.

We are also very happy for the materials in our books to be shared amongst women's communities: to be studied by book groups, discussed in classes, read from in ceremony, quoted on social media...with the following provisos:

- If content from the book is shared in written or spoken form, the book's author and title must be referenced clearly.

- The only person fully qualified to teach the material from any of our titles is the author of the book itself. There are no accredited teachers of this work. Please do not make claims of this sort.

- If you are creating a course devoted to the content of one of our books, its title and author must be clearly acknowledged on all promotional material (posters, websites, social media posts).

- The book's cover may be used in promotional materials or social media posts. The cover art is copyright of the artist and has been licensed exclusively for this book. Any element of the book's cover or font may not be used in branding your own marketing materials when teaching the content of the book, or content very similar to the original book.

- No more than two double page spreads, or four single pages of any book may be photocopied as teaching materials.

We are delighted to offer a 20% discount of over five copies going to one address. You can order these on our webshop, or email us. If you require further clarification, email us at: info@womancraftpublishing.com

ALSO FROM WOMANCRAFT

Medicine Woman:
Reclaiming the Soul of Healing

Lucy H. Pearce

This audacious questioning of the current medical system's ability to deal with the modern epidemic of chronic illness, combines a raw personal memoir of sickness and healing, woven through with voices of dozens of other long-term sick women of the world and a feminine cultural critique that digs deep into the roots of patriarchal medicine. Pearce takes us from its ancient Greek roots, through the influences of the Enlightenment and Christianity, the wholesale destruction of the wise woman tradition and Western colonial destruction of native medicines to the current technocratic, capitalist model of medicine.

She of the Sea

Lucy H. Pearce

A lyrical exploration of the call of the sea and the depth of our connection to it, rooted in the author's personal experience living on the coast of the Celtic Sea, in Ireland.

This book spans from coastal plants to the colour blue, pebbles to prayer, via shapeshifting and suicidal ideation, erosion and immersion, cold water swimming and water birth, seaweed and cyanotypes, from Japanese freedivers and Celtic sea goddesses, selkies to surfing, and mermaids to Mary.

She of the Sea is a strange and wonderful deep dive into the inner sea and the Feminine, exploring where the real and the magical, the salty and the sacred meet, within and without, and what implications this has for us as both individuals... and a species in these tumultuous times.

Home to Her: Walking the Transformative Path of the Sacred Feminine

Liz Childs Kelly

A journey, personal and collective, through time and place, to remember and reconnect with the lost and stolen wisdom of the Sacred Feminine, an ancient Divine force known intimately by ancestral peoples around the world. While in some cultures She remains a vibrant, living force, in the West Her wisdom and traditions have been lost or buried by patriarchal religions and traditions.

Walking with Persephone: A Journey of Midlife Descent and Renewal

Molly Remer

Midlife can be a time of great change – inner and outer: a time of letting go of the old, burnout and disillusionment. But how do we journey through this? And what can we learn in the process? Molly Remer is our personal guide to the unraveling and reweaving required in midlife. She invites you to take a walk with the goddess Persephone, whose story of descent into the underworld has much to teach us.

Walking with Persephone is a story of devotion and renewal that weaves together personal experiences, insights, observations, and reflections with experiences in practical priestessing, family life, and explorations of the natural world. It advocates opening our eyes to the wonder around us, encouraging the reader to both look within themselves for truths about living, but also to the earth, the air, the sky, the animals, and plants.